Lecture Notes in Statistics

Volume 226

Lecture Notes in Statistics (LNS) includes research work on topics that are more specialized than volumes in Springer Series in Statistics (SSS).

The series editors are currently Peter Bühlmann, Peter Diggle, Ursula Gather, and Scott Zeger. Peter Bickel, Ingram Olkin, and Stephen Fienberg were editors of the series for many years.

Jesús López-Fidalgo

Optimal Experimental Design

A Concise Introduction for Researchers

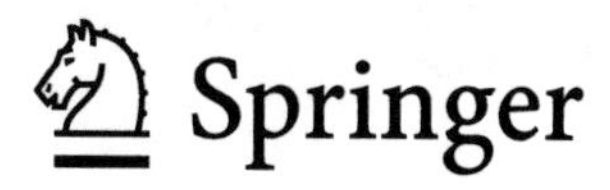

Jesús López-Fidalgo
Institute of Data Science and Artificial
Intelligence
University of Navarre
Pamplona, Spain

ISSN 0930-0325 ISSN 2197-7186 (electronic)
Lecture Notes in Statistics
ISBN 978-3-031-35917-0 ISBN 978-3-031-35918-7 (eBook)
https://doi.org/10.1007/978-3-031-35918-7

Mathematics Subject Classification: 62K05, 62B15, 62B10, 94A15

This Springer imprint is published by the registered company Springer Nature Switzerland AG
The registered company address is: Gewerbestrasse 11, 6330 Cham, Switzerland

Paper in this product is recyclable.

To my parents Jesús and Elvira and my brother Santi

Preface

I have enjoyed very much writing this book. This is very important from a personal point of view, but I believe this is the key of writing something interesting for the readers. One of the main advantages for an optimal experimental design (OED) researcher is that he or she walks around many different topics in statistics and even in some areas of mathematics and other sciences. Thus, designing optimally an experiment may be an objective for any kind of model such as survival analysis or reliability, models with correlated observations, kinetics and compartmental models, mixed models, mixture of distributions, models of mixtures, censoring and potential missing data, model discrimination, mathematical programming... This means one is frequently introduced in a new area without changing the main field of research. Even if the optimal designs are not used at the end this theory, they help to understand more deeply the estimation errors and correlations between them.

The book provides a concise introduction to optimal experimental design theory giving the usual techniques of this field. This introduction wants to be both of help for people starting to work on OED and a reference for all. The book is addressed to researchers or students of statistics or applied mathematics, who have taken up a course in mathematical statistics. As for engineers or other practitioners, this text can also be of use, since appendices include supplementary material on basic measure theory, but they may need to read some practical introduction to measure and integration if they are not very familiar with these matters, e.g., Carter and van Brunt (2000). Otherwise, the procedures in the book can be followed and reproduced even if there is not a deep knowledge of the topic.

An important part of the book deals with what we think are some hot topics for research on OED. For further reading on the area, we may recommend a number of good books with the risk of omitting some relevant ones (Fedorov, 1972; Chernoff, 2000; Silvey, 1980; Pázman, 1986; Shah and Sinha, 1989; Logothetis and Wynn, 1989; Atkinson and Donev, 1992; Pilz, 1993; Pukelsheim, 1993; Rasch and Darius, 1995; Schwabe, 1996; Fedorov and Hackl, 1997; Dette and Studden, 1997; Müller, 1997; Walter and Pronzato, 1997; Liski et al., 2002; Berger and Wong, 2005; Melas, 2006; Atkinson et al., 2007b; Müller, 2007a; Bailey, 2008; Pronzato and Zhigljavsky, 2008; Gibilisco et al., 2009; Berger and Wong, 2009; Rasch et al.,

2010; Goos and Jones, 2011; Fedorov and Leonov, 2013; Kitsos, 2013; Pronzato and Pázman, 2013; Celant and Broniatowski, 2017; Dean et al., 2020) as well as the long series of proceedings of the MODA conferences (Dodge et al., 1988; Müller et al., 1993; Kitsos and Müller, 1995; Atkinson et al., 1998, 2001b; Di Buchianico et al., 2004; López-Fidalgo et al., 2007; Giovanolly et al., 2010; Atkinson et al., 2013; Müller and Atkinson, 2016; Harman et al., 2019; Woods, 2023) and other books of papers (Brown et al., 1985; Flournoy et al., 1998; Atkinson et al., 2001a). We beg pardon to the authors of the books omitted here by ignorance. It is fair to remark that the origin of this theory is in a long paper of a woman, Smith (1918).

The book may be useful to new researchers in OED. Nevertheless, the real examples and the way concepts and results are introduced may be of interest also for different areas of application. Thus, an engineer or a physician may be interested in reading important parts of the book. There are also references to the existing software and web sites for computing designs easily. For instance, pharmacokinetics is a strong area of application for OED. Frequently, the models are derived from differential equations, either ordinary or partial differential equations. If the models can be obtained analytically, the problem of obtaining optimal designs is the usual one. If not, there are cases where the FIM can be obtained explicitly from the system of differential equations. In other cases, some numerical approaches are needed. This area is very much in contact with computer experiments and spatial statistics. Many of the examples in the book consider these type of models.

As mentioned above, the book gives a careful introduction to optimal experimental design in a practical way. It is written with mathematical accuracy in such a way an OED non-specialist statistician can be introduced in the topic appropriately. But at the same time, since the problem is stated from the basis, it can be read by a non-statistician understanding the main ideas and the whole context. Chapter 1 gives a without-formulae introduction and motivation. The chapter ends with some usual criticisms to OED taking advantage of them to provide some hints to use the results properly. Then, Chap. 2 establishes the theory for linear models, concepts, and results, and provides the most important techniques to do research in this area and to compute optimal designs for particular situations. Thus, some typical algorithms are introduced as well as software references.

Chapter 3 is devoted to nonlinear models. The whole theory of OED is beautiful and smooth for linear models. When some constraint is added, the theory has to be adapted in a proper way, usually trough approximations. This is an important challenge and needs to be treated carefully in each particular situation. This chapter introduces nonlinear models in an original way, justifying the theory with elegant arguments for two versions of the exponential family. Section 3.10 provides a deep introduction to another area of much interest nowadays, spatial and temporal statistics where the observations are correlated. Two important problems arise immediately. On the one hand, the approximation of the covariance matrix of the Maximum Likelihood Estimators (MLE) through the inverse of the Fisher Information Matrix (FIM) needs special justification here. On the other hand, from a mathematical point of view, modeling the mean or the variance, if the model is heteroscedastic, has not restrictions at all, but modeling the covariance structure is not an easy task. The covariance structure needs to be positive definite. Some theoretical results provide ways to model practical situations, both under isotropic or anisotropic assumptions.

Chapter 4 provides a thorough revision of Bayesian optimal design, which has not been considered much in introductory books like this one.

The rest of the book is devoted to particular topics of interest as well as recent developments in OED. Some of them are motivated from the criticisms considered in the first chapter. All this is organized in two chapters. Chapter 5 details some hot topics while Chap. 6 provides some real practical examples from the experience of the author. In particular, Chap. 5 starts with computer experiments, which is an emerging area becoming more and more popular (Sect. 5.2). Complex experiments, which are not practicable in real situations, are simulated with complex and slow computer experiments. Thus, a suitable optimal design is needed in this situation. First, a proper objective criterion function has to be introduced. Then, efficient algorithms to compute the designs are crucial here.

In the face of the recent "Big Data" phenomenon, the role of statistics is crucial in extracting maximum information from data, which is the motivation behind the design of experiments. Some of the recent work on this topic will be considered at the end of the book. Thus, Sect. 5.3 gives an introduction of the so called active learning.

In Sect. 5.4, there is a proposal of how optimal experimental design can contribute to the important topic of personalized medicine. Section 5.5 is devoted to designing for discriminating between models when there are several rival models before the data is collected. Different approaches are considered also for non-normal models.

Frequently, in the real life some of the explanatory variables may be designed, but some other have values already known when designing and are not under the control of the experimenter. Sometimes, there is another kind of explanatory variable, which is not under the control of the experimenter, but its values are unknown before the experiment is realized. This situation is considered from the design point of view, which in the later case needs some prior assumptions. Three real examples are provided in Chap. 6.

The word "optimal" in the topic of this book means this theory needs efficient algorithms for computing optimal designs. Actually, this is not an easy task and deserves much work to be done in this direction. During years, traditional algorithms in the area have been used without much ambition to get something better. Recently, there is a good number of publications in this area, which is a good news. For instance, there is some attention on nature-inspired algorithms. They are simple to implement and produce good results in spite of convergence cannot be proved mathematically. Section 5.6 provides a few examples of typical meta-heuristic algorithms.

Chapter 6 provides a few illustrative examples for non-standard situations. An example for correlated observations related to retention of radiation in the human body shows the impact of this topic. Designs for models of mixture of probability distributions have not been considered much in the literature, although they appear to be very useful to model a variety of real situations. The problem of identifiability needs here a deep consideration. Then, computing the FIM, and so optimal designs, becomes a very challenging goal. This is shown as an emerging topic for future research in Sect. 6.2. OED makes sense whenever a variable can be controlled by an experimenter, in a broader sense. It is usual to assume in this case that all the explanatory variables are under control, frequently just one. But in real scenarios, there are mixture of variables under control jointly with uncontrolled variables, whose values come randomly. This is a non-standard situation at all, which is considered in Sects. 6.3, 6.4, and 6.6.

In the real world, some potential censoring emerges frequently. For instance, when the time of an exercise or any other experiment is designed, the exercise may be stopped before reaching the time targeted in the optimal design. This has to be taken into account in advance to compute "optimal expected designs." This is censoring in the explanatory variable under control, but the typical censoring in survival models introduces an important degree of complexity when a design is being optimized before knowing which experimental units are going to be censored. All this is considered in 6.7 and 6.8.

Finally, Appendix provides different mathematical and statistical tools for those interested in the details. Starting by some mathematical concepts and properties related to matrices, an introduction to linear models, probability measure theory, and convex theory is given.

The book contains a number of examples with details in the computations. Additionally, at the end of the main chapters, there are a few exercises. For some of them, the final solution is given so the reader can check whether his or her procedure is correct. Some of them are more complex and hints with more or less details are provided.

In the whole, this brief book wants to be of help for those starting an optimal experimental design adventure.

Acknowledgments

Most of the material of this book comes from years of work on this topic. The work with my former and current PhD students helped me to find the way to make concepts, results an procedures more comprehensible for the reader. Prof. Javier Villarroel helped me to find an elegant proof of the usual claim that approximate designs can be reduced from general probability measures to discrete probability measures before using Caratheodory theorem. Actually, Caratheodory theorem only guarantees that the space of discrete probability measures can be reduced to discrete probability measures with at most $m(m+1)/2$, being m the number of parameters in the model. I believe this is a novel contribution of the book giving a mathematical support of this very welcome property.

Pamplona, Spain Jesús López-Fidalgo

Contents

List of Symbols

A^T:	Transposed of A.
#:	Cardinal of a set.
$\mathbb{R}$:	Real line.
$\mathbb{N}$:	Natural numbers.
∇:	Gradient.
s:	Step in an algorithm.
u_i:	Vector i of the canonical basis.
$\mathrm{Img}(A)$:	Image of the linear function generated by A.
$\mathrm{Ker}(A)$:	Kernel of the linear function generated by A.
E_W or E_π:	Expectation with respect to the distribution of random variable W or pdf π.
Σ_W:	Covariance matrix of a random vector W.
γ:	Confidence coefficient.
y:	Either a particular observation or a vector of n observations.
x:	Vector of explanatory variables.
$f(x)$:	Vector of regressors in a linear model.
$\theta = (\theta_1, \ldots, \theta_m)^T$:	Vector of parameters of a model.
m:	Number of parameters in the model.
η:	Mean model.
$\sigma^2(x)$:	Variance of the response.
$\lambda(x) = \sigma^{-2}(x)$:	Sensitivity function of the response.
$h(y \mid x, \theta)$:	pdf establishing a general statistical model.
$\mathcal{L}$:	Likelihood.
ℓ:	Log-likelihood.
e_i:	Residual for observation i.
ζ:	Experimental design (probability measure).
ξ:	Experimental design (pdf).
ζ_x, ξ_x:	One-point experimental design.
S_ξ:	Design support.

k:	Number of different support points of an experimental design.
χ:	Design space.
p:	Dimension of the design space, that is the number of covariates. It also denotes the weights of an approximate design.
n:	Sample size.
X:	Design matrix.
$X^T X$:	Information matrix of an exact design.
$M(\xi)$ or $M(\xi, \theta)$:	Per observation information matrix of an approximate design.
$M_x = M(\xi_x)$ or $M(\xi_x, \theta)$:	Information matrix at point x.
Φ:	Optimality criterion.
ψ:	Sensitivity function (from the equivalence theorem).
$\xi^\star$:	Optimal design.
μ:	Measure for I-optimality.
$\mathcal{U}(d, \theta, \xi, y)$:	Utility function.
$\mathcal{U}(\xi) = \mathrm{E}_y \max_d \mathrm{E}_\theta [\mathcal{U}(d, \theta, \xi, y)$:	Expected utility function
L:	Loss function.

Chapter 1
Motivating Introduction

1.1 What Is a Statistical Model?

This is not an easy question to answer. Box (1979) used to say "Models, of course, are never true, but fortunately it is only necessary that they be useful." From a simplistic point of view it may be said there are two kinds of mathematical models, either deterministic or statistical models. A deterministic model is completely determined, perhaps with complex formulae or differential equations without an explicit solution available. Frequently the solutions have to be approximated numerically. But all the parameters in the model are assumed completely known, at least from a theoretical point of view. Perhaps the model does not fit perfectly the phenomenon, but there is nothing left to the hazard. When an opportunity is given to randomness a statistical model arises. This means the model is not assumed completely known and therefore something needs to be estimated using data from experiments or sampling, as well as from prior knowledge, previous research, or the intuition of the practitioners. The model can be partially hidden during the whole process or even without an explicit mathematical expression.

Summarizing, a simplistic classification of models may be this,

- Deterministic model: The reality is assumed completely known through it.
- Statistical model: There is a stochastic uncertainty,
  - Classic parametric models.
  - Nonparametric models.
  - Bayesian models, parametric or not.

A very general concept of parametric statistical model is considered in this book. The Bayesian version is also behind it, and it will be rescued later. A model of a particular phenomenon establishes a relationship between at least two variables, for example, the average speed of a car and the consumption of gasoline. In practice, it is quite convenient identifying the dependent and the independent variables to

J. López-Fidalgo, *Optimal Experimental Design*, Lecture Notes in Statistics 226,
https://doi.org/10.1007/978-3-031-35918-7_1

check what is the *response* (*dependent* variables) after some stimulus or experiment (*independent* or *explanatory* variables). If a particular explanatory variable can be controlled by the experimenter, then the different values of the variable to realize the experiments can be designed from an experimental point of view. After performing the experiment, a value of the dependent variable is observed. While the values of the explanatory variable may be assumed fixed, the response (observation) will be different after replicating the same experiment exactly at the same conditions. Thus, the response variable should be considered as a random variable (r.v.).

1.2 Importance of Designing an Experiment

It is important to remark what it is understood by *experiment* in this context. An experiment has the following steps:

1. Fixing some experimental conditions, say particular values of some of the explanatory variables that are under the control of the experimenter. This is the x. Example: a specific temperature and time in a furnace or a particular education program.
2. Take some action with those conditions. Example: put some substance in the furnace during that specific time and temperature.
3. Measure some response when the action has finished. Example: density of the resulting substance after been in the furnace. This is the y.

It is worth to say that some explanatory variables are not under control and therefore they cannot be fixed. Then we refer to observational data instead of experimental data.

This is a classic example to show the importance of designing appropriately the experimentation. We have to estimate the weight of two objects using a traditional scale with two plates, and the budget is just enough for two weights. We may assume that each estimation of a weight has a Gaussian error, ε, with mean 0 and constant variance σ^2. Thus, $y = P + \varepsilon$, where the actual weight is the parameter P to be estimated and the observed weight in the scale is y. Given these conditions and without much thinking, the typical plan (design) of experimentation would be weighing each object one after the other (Fig. 1.1) to estimate the two weights, $\hat{P}_A$ and $\hat{P}_B$.

It is not difficult to see that the Maximum Likelihood Estimator (MLE) is $\hat{P}_A = y_1$ and $\hat{P}_B = y_2$, with standard errors σ. Moreover, both estimators are independent. But, taking into account the assumption of constant variance, the standard error can

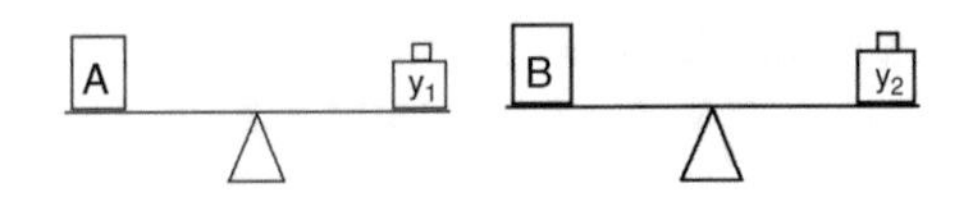

Fig. 1.1 Classical design

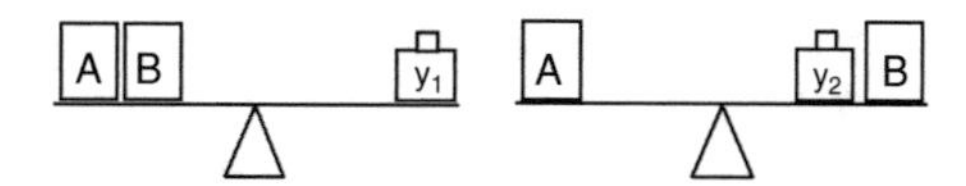

Fig. 1.2 Optimal design

be lowered down using both objects in each weigh. This can be done weighing first the sum of the weights and then the weight difference (Fig. 1.2).

Now the MLEs are $\hat{P}_A = \frac{y_1+y_2}{2}$ and $\hat{P}_B = \frac{y_1-y_2}{2}$ with standard error $\sigma/\sqrt{2}$, which means an important reduction. One may say that this is wonderful, but the estimators seem to be dependent now since both include the same observations. A simple computation shows they are actually uncorrelated and therefore independent,

$$\text{cov}(\hat{P}_A, \hat{P}_B) = \{\text{cov}(y_1, y_1) - \text{cov}(y_1, y_2) + \text{cov}(y_1, y_2) - \text{cov}(y_2, y_2)\}/4 = 0,$$

where "cov" stands for the covariance.

This example is quite illustrative to show the usefulness of thinking before acting, that is, searching for the best experiment. Thus, a good experimental design helps to saving time, money, and risk and frequently allows for a correct statistical analysis of the data.

Basic Principles for an Experimental Design

- *Randomization* legitimates all the statistical analyses, which are based in the laws of randomness. Parametric statistical models are random (stochastic) models where observations are considered random variables with a probability distribution partially known. This allows computation of probabilities in the fitting of the models. The Central Limit Theorem allows also approximating some probabilities, again under typical random assumptions. Thus, the error can be measured and controlled. To do this the data have to be taken in a random way; otherwise, the probability distribution assumptions may be wrong and so the computations. There is a story from Ronald Fisher and Miss Bristol that illustrates well this idea. She was supposed to recognize whether in a cup of tea the milk was added before, say milk with tea, or after the tea, say tea with milk. Fisher challenged her to a trial where in four cups of tea the milk was added before the tea and four where the milk was added after. She went to other room while the experiment was prepared. When the eight cups were carefully filled in that way, one of the students put them in a disordered way. Then Fisher made the remark that this is not a random disposition because random means any disposition of the cups has the same probability to be chosen. Thus, a disposition with all the four cups of milk with tea offered at the beginning has the same probability as offering them in positions, say 1, 4, 5, and 7. The set of "disordered" cups contains the latter but not the former one and many other "symmetric" distributions. These probabilities are used in the fitting of the model that we call sometimes "statistical analysis" and then the error in the results may follow.

- *Replication* of the same experiments gives the chance of measuring the variability of the observations, which is crucial to make inferences and check whether there is a significant extra variability introduced by the explanatory variables or not. Replicate a particular experiment is realizing it again in an independent way, preserving all the conditions as equal as possible. For instance, a chemical reaction is repeated again with the same concentration of the substrate, same temperature, but cleaning all the material carefully to avoid any dependence.
- *Repeated measurements* are a completely different concept of the previous one since two measurements of the same subject are observed, for example, the response to a stimulus is measured in same person before and after drinking alcohol.
- *Blocking* means basically introducing nuisance variables (block factors) in the model to eliminate their influence in the response. Thus, the model can estimate properly the actual effect of the variables of interest. The original example comes from agriculture where the field is divided into different parts (blocks) to avoid the effect of differences in fertility in different locations.

1.3 The Statistical Procedure from the Beginning to the End

We may say that statistics consists in fitting a mathematical model to the reality, controlling the error or discrepancy between model and reality. The whole process can be described as follows:

- Established the real problem to be solved, that is, what we want to prove.
- Select a model, for example, a linear model,

$$\mathrm{E}(y \mid x) = f^T(x)\theta, \; Var(y \mid x) = \sigma^2,$$

  where y the response variable (with variance σ^2), x the vector of explanatory variables, f continuous with components linearly independent, and $\theta = (\theta_1, \ldots, \theta_m)^T$ a vector of parameters to be estimated.
- Select an experimental condition x_1 on a *design space* χ. The homologous for observational data would be choosing at random a subject and measuring all the variables we want, for example, doing a survey. This one is not the aim of this book.
- Perform the experiment and observe the response y_1.
- Repeat the process for the experimental conditions $x_2, \ldots, x_n$ obtaining responses $y_2, \ldots, y_n$.
- Estimate the parameters $\theta_1, \ldots, \theta_m, \sigma^2$ and make inferences with them such as comparing them to zero.
- Interpret and communicate the results and make decisions.

1.4 Criticisms and Rejoinders

Although the classic theory of experimental design is well-known, this is not the case when the word "optimal" is added. The classic experimental design is looking for good designs, studying their properties and trying to generate some types of designs. Meanwhile, the optimal design theory aims the best possible design, mainly from a regression setup, including somehow classic designs as in Dorta-Guerra et al. (2008). The word "optimal" introduces some typical criticism in the sense that it takes sometimes to extremal solutions. Some criticisms come from practitioners, some from statisticians. One of the main tasks of the statisticians is to convince the practitioner they need to design their experimentation correctly and efficiently apart from doing the correct statistical analysis. The aim of this section is to offer a simple introduction to the topic through these critical views.

1.4.1 Model Dependence

One of the main criticisms to the optimal experimental design (OED) theory is that a model has to be selected a priory without any data yet. This is a deeper problem that it seems to be at the first sight. Frequently there is a strong dependence between the model and the optimal design. Thus, a design may be rather good for a particular model and pathetic for a different one, which may finally be proved much better for the actual data.

Rejoinder Box used to write frequently statements like: "Models, of course, are never true, but fortunately it is only necessary that they be useful" (Box, 1979). This idea does not solve the problem mentioned in the last paragraph but stresses the truth that this is not only a problem of designing an experiment. In any case the experiment needs to be designed before having the observations and the problem has to be undertaken with the tools at hand at that moment. In practice, there is always some experience or retrospective data one can trust. There are also the intuitions of the practitioner. Even some models are analytically derived, for example, solving a differential equation system.

Moreover, there is a particular interest nowadays in developing optimality criteria to discriminate between rival models (e.g., López-Fidalgo et al., 2007b, 2008b) when there are several candidates to be the best model. There is also a more global point of view related to search for optimal design for maximizing the power of lack-of-fit tests (Wiens, 1991; O'Brien, 1995; Bischoff & Miller, 2006; Wiens, 2019).

1.4.2 Information Matrix for Nonlinear Models

The optimal design theory is clean for linear models, but most of the models used in practice are not linear in different ways. The theory, including the equivalence theorem, still applies for a variety of nonlinear models, but the information matrix will depend on the "no yet" estimated parameters.

Rejoinder This is not a negligible objection at all, but there are several reasonable ways to tackle the problem:

- Locally Φ-optimal designs may be computed depending on nominal values of the parameters. Some times explicit optimal designs may be given depending on generic values of the parameter, but usually numerical computations are needed, and some explicit numerical values of the parameters have to be used in the computations. In any case, a sensitivity analysis should be carried out to be sure the design is not going to change much with the possible errors in the choice of the parameters.
- Going further with the last idea minimax designs may be computed to be safer.
- An approach of great current interest is the adaptive design idea (e.g., Moler et al., 2006), where at each step the designs used the observations obtained previously. The parameters are estimated in each step and thus the dependence becomes less and less important along the process.
- Another typical approach to this problem is the use of some kind of Bayesian designs.

1.4.3 Criterion Selection

As it was pointed out in the Introduction, there is a number of different criteria, sometimes even parametric classes of them (see, e.g., Rodríguez-Díaz & López-Fidalgo, 2003) pursuing different aims.

Rejoinder In practice, a few optimality criteria are really used and the choice of one of them is not a big deal. Moreover, the original equivalence theorem, much more restricted than the general one, proved the equivalence (so the name) of D-optimality and a criterion to minimize the variance of the predictions (G-optimality). This means the optimal designs are not always so far for different criteria. Even more, under some conditions there exist designs universally optimal (Harman, 2008). Nevertheless, if there is interest in different criteria producing different optimal designs, compound criteria must be used to come to a compromise for a desirable design (Cook & Wong, 1994).

1.4.4 Controversy of Exact Versus Approximate Designs

Approximate designs are quite convenient from a theoretical and computational point of view. But to be implemented in practice, a kind of rounding-off is needed with the corresponding loss of efficiency in the design. On the contrary, exact designs are practicable but of very difficult computation. Box has never accepted the use of the approximate designs introduced by Kiefer (1959).

Rejoinder This controversy should not affect the development of the theory. After years of experience in the area, it may be said that exact designs are needed, and less difficult to compute, for small sample sizes (Pukelsheim & Rieder, 1992; Imhof & Wong, 2000). For large samples the approximate designs may be rounded off in an efficient way.

1.4.5 Frequently, Optimal Designs Demand Extreme Conditions

A typical situation in statistics is that extreme conditions in the experiments offer, “theoretically,” more information to make decisions. But this may be non-affordable, toxic, dangerous, or just awful for the practitioners. Even more, if the optimal design reduces to a few points, less than what they would like, they would reject any use of it.

Rejoinder This is absolutely true and the statistician has to be very careful with this aspect. Frequently, the optimal design has to be considered as a reference to measure the efficiency of the designs the experimenters use in practice or to choose the best among a class of designs they like. On the other hand, the criteria used may restrict the search to a class of designs to preserve the requirements of the practitioners.

1.4.6 Difficult Computation

Computation of optimal designs is not an easy task in general. As a matter of fact, the search for optimal designs frequently restricts to one-dimensional models, although some work has been performed with more complex models (Garcet-Rodríguez et al., 2008).

Rejoinder There is an increasing interest in developing good algorithms to compute designs, either exact or approximate designs (see, e.g., Martin-Martin et al., 2007 or Harman et al., 2020). One may think the people working on optimal design must be good in optimization. They are not bad, but they are not specialists in the topic. At the same time, people in optimization are sometimes far from statistics and even more from experimental designs. Therefore, there is a need of more cooperation between them.

1.4.7 Scale Problem

Some criteria are not invariant with respect to reparameterizations. This means that the scale of a parameter may be much bigger than the scale of another parameter in the model, causing different magnitudes of the variances of their estimators. Therefore, the criterion may not pay attention enough to the small variance in magnitude, but equally important in the inference. This is the case of A-optimality, among other criteria.

Rejoinder This problem requires special care and some standardization of the criteria. Different solutions have been given to this problem. For instance, standardized optimality criteria by the efficiencies of each parameter (Dette, 1997) produce similar final efficiencies for estimating each parameter of the model regardless the magnitude of the variances of the estimators. Another possible standardization is by the coefficient of variation (López-Fidalgo & Rivas-López, 2007; López-Fidalgo et al., 2007a). This last adds a dependence on the parameters that it is not so relevant for nonlinear models since here the dependence on the parameters is unavoidable. For D-optimality, the most popular criterion, based on the determinant of the Fisher Information Matrix (FIM), the standardization is not necessary.

Chapter 2
Optimal Design Theory for Linear Models

2.1 The Linear Model

Let y be the response (a univariate or multivariate random variable or vector) and assume x is a vector of explanatory variables (predictors), which can be controlled by the experimenter. A *linear model* trying to describe the relationship between y and the values of x can be described as

$$y = \theta^T f(x) + \varepsilon, \tag{2.1}$$

where $\theta^T = (\theta_1, \ldots, \theta_m)$ is the vector of unknown parameters to be estimated, $f^T(x) = (f_1(x), \ldots, f_m(x))$ is a vector of known linearly independent continuous functions, and x is an experimental condition (nonrandom), which can be chosen on a *design space*, χ, a compact set on a Euclidean space, typically an interval or a finite set. The response y is assumed normal with mean $\mathrm{E}(y) = \theta^T f(x)$, that is, $\mathrm{E}(\varepsilon) = 0$ and constant variance $\mathrm{var}(y) = \mathrm{var}(\varepsilon) = \sigma^2$.

Thus, a linear model assumes independence, normality, homoscedasticity, as well as linearity of the mean with respect to the parameters.

Example 2.1 These are examples of linear models assuming independence, normality, and homoscedasticity:

1. Simple linear regression: $y = \theta_0 + \theta_1 x + \varepsilon,\ f^T(x) = (1, x),\ x \in \chi = [a, b]$.
2. Multiple linear regression without intercept: $y = \theta_1 x_1 + \theta_2 x_2 + \theta_3 x_3 + \varepsilon,\ f^T(x) = x = (x_1, x_2, x_3),\ x \in \chi = [a_1, b_1] \times [a_2, b_2] \times [a_3, b_3]$.
3. Quadratic regression: $y = \theta_0 + \theta_1 x + \theta_2 x^2 + \varepsilon,\ f^T(x) = (1, x, x^2),\ x \in \chi = [a, b]$.

J. López-Fidalgo, *Optimal Experimental Design*, Lecture Notes in Statistics 226,
https://doi.org/10.1007/978-3-031-35918-7_2

4. Analysis of the Variance (ANOVA) (one-way, three levels):

$$y = \theta_0 + \theta_1 x_1 + \theta_2 x_2 + \varepsilon,\ f^T(x_1, x_2) = (1, x_1, x_2),\ x = (x_1, x_2) \in \chi$$
$$= \{(0, 1), (1, 0), (1, 1)\}.$$

The typical matrix form of a linear model is now adapted to this notation. Assume the experiment is realized n times at n *experimental conditions* $x_1, x_2, \ldots, x_n$. Let $y_1, y_2, \ldots, y_n$ be the corresponding independent outcomes (responses) and $\varepsilon_1, \varepsilon_2, \ldots, \varepsilon_n$ the random errors,

$$X = \begin{pmatrix} f_1(x_1) & \cdots & f_m(x_1) \\ \cdots & \cdots & \cdots \\ \cdots & f_j(x_i) & \cdots \\ \cdots & \cdots & \cdots \\ f_1(x_n) & \cdots & f_m(x_n) \end{pmatrix},\ Y = \begin{pmatrix} y_1 \\ \vdots \\ y_i \\ \vdots \\ y_n \end{pmatrix},\ \mathcal{E} = \begin{pmatrix} \varepsilon_1 \\ \vdots \\ \varepsilon_i \\ \vdots \\ \varepsilon_n \end{pmatrix}.$$

Then (2.1) can be expressed as

$$Y = X\theta + \mathcal{E}.$$

For linear models the Least Squares Estimators (LSE) coincide with the Maximum Likelihood Estimators and, by the Gauss-Markov theorem, with the Best Linear Unbiased Estimators (BLUEs),

$$\hat{\theta} = (X^T X)^{-1} X^T Y.$$

The covariance matrix of the parameter estimators is then

$$\Sigma_{\hat{\theta}} = \sigma^2 (X^T X)^{-1}. \tag{2.2}$$

The confidence ellipsoid of the parameters comes from this matrix,

$$(\hat{\theta} - \theta)^T (X^T X)^{-1} (\hat{\theta} - \theta) \le m F_{m,n-m,\gamma} S_R^2,$$

where $F_{m,n-m,\gamma}$ stands for the quantile γ (confidence level) of the F-distribution, $S_R^2 = \frac{1}{n-m} \sum_{i=1}^n e_i^2$ is the residual variance, and $E = Y - X\hat{\theta} = (e_1, \ldots, e_n)^T$ are the residuals.

The confidence band for the mean at a particular value is

$$y_{m,i} = \hat{y}_{m,i} \pm t_{n-m,\frac{\gamma+1}{2}} S_R \sqrt{X_i^T (X^T X)^{-1} X_i},$$

where X_i^T is the i-th row of X.

The individual prediction band for a particular response at specific conditions is

$$y_i = \hat{y}_i \pm t_{n-m,\frac{\gamma+1}{2}} S_R \sqrt{1 + X_i^T (X^T X)^{-1} X_i}.$$

More details about this can be found in Appendix B.

2.2 From Exact to Approximate Designs

If the reader wants to understand better what follows there is an introduction to measure theory is provided in Appendix F. Otherwise, the reader can go on with an intuitive idea of probability measures and their properties.

An *exact design* of size n is just a collection of points $x_1, x_2, \ldots, x_n$, where the experiment is being realized. They are chosen by the practitioner from the design space χ. It will be called ξ_n.

Example 2.2 Revisiting some of the previous models, these are possible exact designs:

1. For $\chi = [0, 1]$, these are possible designs of size 6: $0, 0.2, 0.4, 0.6, 0.8, 1$ or $0, 0, 0, 1, 1, 1$.
4. For $\chi = \{(0, 1), (1, 0), (1, 1)\}$, possible designs are $(0, 1), (1, 0), (1, 1)$ (size 3) or $(0, 1), (0, 1), (1, 0), (1, 0), (1, 1)$ (size 5).

Since some of the points may be repeated, a finite support probability measure can be defined on χ with probabilities $\xi(x) = \frac{n_x}{n}$, where n_x is the number of times x appears in the design.

Example 2.3

1. For $0, 0, 0, 1, 1, 1$; the probability mass function is defined as $\xi(0) = \xi(1) = 1/2$ and $\xi(x) = 0$ for any $x \neq 0, 1$.
4. For $(0, 1), (0, 1), (1, 0), (1, 0), (1, 1)$; the design is defined as $\xi[(0, 1)] = \xi[(1, 0)] = 2/5$ and $\xi[(1, 1)] = 1/5$.

This idea suggests a "wicked" mathematical perversion of extending the concept of experimental design to any probability measure. This idea came from Kiefer (1974) and it used to be a controversial topic that George Box and others never have liked. It is not just a beautiful theoretical extension. This definition gives a nice theorem, which allows one to check whether a specific design is optimal or not according to a particular criterion. This also provides a tool to build algorithms for computing optimal designs and bounds for the goodness of a particular design. Thus, a probability measure ζ on the Borel field generated by the open sets of χ will be called *approximate design*. The convex set of all approximate experimental designs will be denoted by Ξ. If the measure is discrete or absolutely continuous with respect to Lebesgue measure, ξ will denote the probability mass function or the probability density function (pdf), respectively.

In practice, for a discrete measure, ξ, the experimenter has to perform n_i experiments at each particular value of the design, say x_i, in such a way $\sum_i n_i = n$. Thus, if the sample size is going to be n, then "approximately" $n\xi(x_i)$ experiments will be realized at x_i. The appropriate rounding-off procedure is not so simple. The nearest integer system does not necessarily lead to the best exact optimal design among the possible rounded-off designs. Pukelsheim and Rieder (1992) provided an interesting discussion about this topic. In Casero-Alonso and López-Fidalgo (2015), there is one example where an approximate optimal design is a one-point design at $x = 1$ while the optimal exact design of any size $n \geq 2$ asks for realizing $n - 1$ experiments at $x = 1$ and just one at $x = 0$. In this case no rounding-off procedure applied to the approximate optimal design leads to the optimal exact design.

As regards the exact versus approximate designs controversy, we may say that a proper compromise gives a reasonable solution (see, e.g., Imhof et al. (2001) for some examples). In particular, if the sample size is large, any rounding-off procedure leads to a quite good exact design. Thus, in this case one can take advantage of this useful theory for computing approximate designs. Otherwise, if n is small then the impact of the rounding-off may be quite important. It is important to stress that the approximate design does not depend on the experiment size n. Thus, when different approximate designs are compared, this is done assuming that the same number of experiments are going to be realized.

The support of a probability measure ζ, say S_ζ, is a precise notion of the "possible" points of the space χ for that probability. It is defined to be the largest subset of χ for which every open neighborhood of every point of the set has positive measure. In theory any probability measure is a candidate design, but we will see that we can restrict the search to finite designs, easier to realize in practice. The *support of a design* with finite support, $S_\xi = \{x : \xi(x) > 0\}$, will be the set of points of χ with positive masses.

2.3 The Information Matrix

The covariance matrix of the estimators of θ is (2.2). For an exact design of size n

$$X^T X = \sum_{i=1}^{n} f(x_i) f^T(x_i) = \sum_{i=1}^{k} n_i f(x_i) f^T(x_i) = n \sum_{i=1}^{k} \xi(x_i) f(x_i) f^T(x_i)$$

is the so-called *information matrix* (apart from σ^2). Here it was assumed that there are k different points in the design, and without loss of generality it may be assumed they are the first k in the list. Then, n_i is the number of replicates of the experiment at $x_i, i = 1, \ldots, k$. Using this expression, the information matrix can be generalized for an approximate design, ζ,

$$M(\zeta) = \int_{\chi} f(x) f^T(x) \zeta(dx).$$

If ζ is discrete and ξ is the probability function associated, then

$$M(\zeta) \equiv M(\xi) = \sum_{x \in \chi} f(x) f^T(x) \xi(x)$$

If ζ is absolutely continuous with respect to the Lebesgue measure, there exists a density (pdf), ξ, such that

$$M(\zeta) \equiv M(\xi) = \int_{\chi} f(x) f^T(x) \xi(x) dx$$

Symbols ζ and ξ will be used indistinctly in the notation for these cases. Properly, this is the "per observation" information matrix. This matrix coincides with the Fisher Information Matrix (FIM) as will be shown with more detail for nonlinear models. We will refer to this matrix hereafter as the FIM. For an approximate design, the covariance matrix is then $\sigma^2 n^{-1} M^{-1}(\zeta)$.

By construction the information matrix is symmetric and nonnegative definite as the covariance matrix is. Let $\mathcal{M}$ be the set of all the information matrices. This is a compact and convex set within the cone of nonnegative definite symmetric matrices within the Euclidean space of dimension $m(m+1)/2$ (see Appendix F.4 for details). Hereafter the superscript $+$ in any set will refer to the nonsingular information matrices. Any FIM is a convex combination, at least in the limit, of information matrices associated to one-point designs, that is, a Dirac measure with all the mass at one point, say x_0,

$$\xi_{x_0}(x) = \begin{cases} 1 \text{ if } x = x_0 \\ 0 \text{ if } x \neq x_0 \end{cases}$$

and its information matrix is $M_{x_0} = f(x_0) f^T(x_0)$. Caratheodory's theorem states that any point of a convex hull of a set in a Euclidean space is a convex combination of no more than the dimension plus one points of the original set. If $\mathcal{M}$ is restricted to matrices coming from finite support designs,

$$\xi = \begin{Bmatrix} x_1 & x_2 & \ldots & x_k \\ p_1 & p_2 & \ldots & p_k \end{Bmatrix},$$

all the theory applies in the same way as for probability distributions. Then the application of this theorem here states that for any information matrix there is always a design with at most $\frac{1}{2}m(m+1)+1$ different points in its support associated to this matrix. Moreover, if the matrix is on the boundary, then the design has no more than $\frac{1}{2}m(m+1)$ different points in its support. More details are given in Appendix F.4 justifying this result for the whole set of designs as general probability measures. As far as the author knows, this proof has not been given before explicitly.

Example 2.4 Let a simple linear regression model be

$$y = \theta_0 + \theta_1 x + \varepsilon,\ x \in \chi = [0, 1],\ f(x) = (1, x)^T.$$

Consider a particular approximate design

$$\xi = \left\{ \begin{matrix} 0 & 0.5 & 1 \\ 0.2 & 0.4 & 0.4 \end{matrix} \right\}.$$

The associated information matrix is then

$$\begin{aligned} M(\xi) &= \sum_{i=1}^{3} \begin{pmatrix} 1 & x_i \\ x_i & x_i^2 \end{pmatrix} p_i \\ &= \begin{pmatrix} 1 & 0 \\ 0 & 0 \end{pmatrix} 0.2 + \begin{pmatrix} 1 & 0.5 \\ 0.5 & 0.25 \end{pmatrix} 0.4 + \begin{pmatrix} 1 & 1 \\ 1 & 1 \end{pmatrix} 0.4 \\ &= \begin{pmatrix} 1 & 0.6 \\ 0.6 & 0.5 \end{pmatrix}. \end{aligned}$$

Let us assume there is budget just for $n = 12$ experiments and the design ξ wants to be performed. Thus, about $0.2 \times 12 = 2.4$ experiments have to be realized at 0, $0.4 \times 12 = 4.8$ at 0.5, and about $0.4 \times 12 = 4.8$ at 1. For this, there are three reasonable possible methods of rounding-off:

1. Design $\xi_{12}^{\star}$: 2, 5, and 5 experiments at 0, 0.5, and 1, respectively.
2. Design $\xi_{12}^{\star\star}$: 3, 4, and 5 experiments at 0, 0.5, and 1, respectively.
3. Design $\xi_{12}^{\star\star\star}$: 3, 5, and 4 experiments at 0, 0.5, and 1, respectively.

It is not as simple as the usual rounding-off. Although (1) is the usual rounding-off procedure, options (2) or (3) may be preferable according to a particular objective. We will see how the goodness of each rounded design can be measured.

2.4 Optimality Criteria

For a linear model the inverse of the FIM is proportional to the covariance matrix, which contains the errors of the estimators of the parameters of the model. Therefore, it is natural to look for experimental designs minimizing some aspect of the inverse of the FIM. Actually, this is a multi-objective problem leading to a number of different criteria with different mathematical and statistical meanings.

A criterion function Φ will be a real function defined on the set of all possible designs,

$$\Phi : \Xi \to \mathbb{R} \cup \{+\infty\},$$

or else, in a more tractable manner, defined on the set of the information matrices,

$$\Phi : \mathcal{M} \to \mathbb{R} \cup \{+\infty\}.$$

In either case a Φ- *optimal design*, say $\zeta^\star$ or $\xi^\star$, will be a design minimizing the criterion function Φ. The superscript $\star$ will usually refer in the future to optimal designs. A criterion may be either *global* if the whole model parameters are of interest or *partial* if the efficient estimation of some of the parameters does not matter.

For the first definition, a criterion is said *convex* if

$$\Phi[(1-\epsilon)\zeta + \epsilon\zeta'] \leq (1-\epsilon)\Phi(\zeta) + \epsilon\Phi(\zeta'),\ \epsilon \in [0, 1].$$

For the second definition,

$$\Phi[(1-\epsilon)M(\xi)] + \epsilon M(\xi')] \leq (1-\epsilon)\Phi[M(\xi)] + \epsilon\Phi[M(\xi')],\ \epsilon \in [0, 1].$$

The first definition is more general and considers important criteria not directly related to information matrices. This is the case of some criteria for discrimination between models.

The second definition has to be considered properly as a function of M^{-1}, which is the objective, and it is usually assumed that Φ is bounded from below and nonincreasing with respect to the Loewner ordering. That is, if $M \leq N$, that is, $N - M$ is nonnegative definite, then $\Phi(M) \geq \Phi(N)$. It may be proved that this ordering means a universal ordering of the information matrices for better estimating the parameters of the model. Specifically (Pázman, 1986, chapter III),

(i) Let c be a vector in $\mathbb{R}^m$ is such that $c^T\theta$ is estimable for a design ξ. Then Var$(c^T\hat{\theta})$ is proportional to $c^t M^-(\xi)c$, where superscript $-$ stands for a pseudo-inverse or generalized inverse (g-inverse) of a matrix, which generalizes the concept of inverse matrix to any matrix, singular or even rectangular. Appendix A states its definition and some properties.

(ii) If $M(\xi) \geq M(\xi')$ then $c^t M^-(\xi)c \leq c^t M^-(\xi')c$ for every $c \in \text{Img}[M(\xi')]$, where $\text{Img}[M(\xi')]$ is the image of the linear function generated by $M(\xi')$ (see Appendix A). This is a very important result since the Loewner ordering on the information matrices means the estimator of any linear combination for a design ξ is not worse than another design ξ' if $M(\xi) \geq M(\xi')$ is satisfied. Thus, a nondecreasing condition has to be considered for any objective function looking at the best design in some sense.

To simplify the notation it will be written $\Phi(\xi)$ instead of $\Phi[M(\xi)]$ if there is not possible confusion. Obviously, there is an equivalent theory assuming nondecreasing and concave functions instead.

2.4.1 General Properties for Global Criteria

Let Φ be a global criterion. Since a global criterion is interested in all the parameters of the model, then the information matrix has to be nonsingular to have the chance to estimate all the parameters. Since any design with less than m different points gives a singular information matrix, any Φ-optimal design has at least m points in its support.

A criterion function Φ is strictly decreasing if $N \leq M$ and $N \neq M$ imply that $\Phi(N) > \Phi(M)$. This double condition is less strong than $N < M$ and it is still appropriate for this definition (see, e.g., Pázman, 1986, Proposition III.3; or Fedorov & Leonov, 2013, Proposition 9.1).

Proposition 2.1 *For strictly decreasing criteria there is always an optimal design with no more than $m(m+1)/2$ points in its support.*

Proof In this case the optimal must be in the boundary. This reduces the dimension in one unit, $m(m+1)/2 - 1$, and using Caratheodory's theorem on the boundary, the limit of different points is then $m(m+1)/2$. □

Remark 2.1

1. If $\sigma^2(x)$ is not constant, the whole theory is applicable for

$$\tilde{f}(x) = f(x)/\sigma(x).$$

   Thus, for simplicity and without loss of generality we will assume $\sigma(x) = 1$ hereafter.
2. If the observations are correlated and Σ_Y is the covariance matrix, then the information matrix, $X^T \Sigma_Y^{-1} X$, is not additive anymore in the sense that it is not a sum in which each term depends just on one experiment as is the case for uncorrelated observations, typically $n \sum_i \frac{n_i}{n} X_i X_i^T$. In the last expression the weights $\frac{n_i}{n}$ define a mass probability function, and the experimental design extension to probability measures makes sense. This extension of the definition

of an experimental design as a probability measure cannot be done for correlated observations. Therefore, just exact designs will be used in this context.
3. For strictly convex criteria the optimal information matrix is unique, although different designs may take to the same optimal information matrix.

2.4.2 *Efficiency*

A criterion is said *inverse positive homogeneous* if

$$\Phi(\delta M) = \frac{1}{\delta}\Phi(M), \quad \delta > 0.$$

This is important to interpret the statistical goodness of a particular design. Let Φ be any criterion function. The Φ- *efficiency* of a design ξ is

$$\mathrm{eff}_{\Phi}[M(\xi)] = \Phi[M(\xi^{\star})]/\Phi[M(\xi)],$$

where $\xi^{\star}$ is a Φ-optimal design. The efficiency is frequently multiplied by 100 and reported in percentage. The efficiency is always between 0 and 1, and it has a clear and useful mathematical meaning in the context of optimization. The higher the efficiency, the better a design is with respect to the objective function. For a general objective function this interpretation is not linear in the sense that and efficiency of 90% does not necessarily duplicates the preference of an efficiency of 45%. Positive homogeneity gives precisely a statistical interpretation very easy to understand for any practitioner.

If the criterion is inverse positive homogeneous and n experiments are being realized, then the efficiency of an approximate design measures actually the efficiency of the covariance matrices for the corresponding exact design associated,

$$\mathrm{eff}_{\Phi}[M(\xi)] = \frac{\Phi[M(\xi^{*})]}{\Phi[M(\xi)]} = \frac{\Phi(\sigma^{-2} n \Sigma_{\hat{\theta}}^{\star -1})}{\Phi(\sigma^{-2} n \Sigma_{\hat{\theta}}^{-1})} = \frac{\sigma^{2} n^{-1} \Phi(\Sigma_{\hat{\theta}}^{\star -1})}{\sigma^{2} n^{-1} \Phi(\Sigma_{\hat{\theta}}^{-1})} = \frac{\Phi(\Sigma_{\hat{\theta}}^{\star -1})}{\Phi(\Sigma_{\hat{\theta}}^{-1})}.$$

The third equality comes from the homogeneity.

The question is now how many experiments, say $n^{\star}$, the optimal experimental design ξ^{*} needs to perform as well as ξ with n experiments. Let us assume the efficiency of ξ is $\gamma \leq 1$, then

$$1 = \frac{\Phi(\Sigma_{\hat{\theta}}^{\star -1})}{\Phi(\Sigma_{\hat{\theta}}^{-1})} = \frac{\sigma^{2} n^{\star -1} \Phi[M(\xi^{*})]}{\sigma^{2} n^{-1} \Phi[M(\xi)]} = \frac{n^{\star -1}}{n^{-1}}\gamma.$$

Therefore, just $n^{\star} = \gamma n$ observations would be enough with ξ^{*} to get the same value of the objective function. In particular, if the efficiency is 50%, then the design

ξ needs to double the total number of observations to perform as well as the optimal design $\xi^\star$.

Some of the most popular optimality criteria will be considered in what follows.

2.4.3 D-optimality

D-optimality is the most popular criterion, likely because it is easier to manage than other criteria and it has an interesting statistical meaning. Wald (1943) introduced this criterion. Kiefer and Wolfowitz (1960) called it D-optimality and they extended it to a general regression model. Fedorov (1972) and Wynn (1970) gave a celebrated algorithm for computing D-optimal designs based on the equivalence theorem. Silvey and Titterington (1973) provided a geometric argument for the construction of D-optimal designs.

The goal of this criterion is to minimize the determinant of the inverse of the information matrix, equivalently maximize the determinant of the information matrix. The criterion function is usually defined as follows:

$$\Phi_D[M(\xi)] = \begin{cases} \log\det M^{-1}(\xi) = -\log\det M(\xi) & \text{if } \det M(\xi) \neq 0, \\ \infty & \text{if } \det M(\xi) = 0. \end{cases}$$

But to have a homogeneous function, an equivalent definition is

$$\Phi_D[M(\xi)] = \begin{cases} \det M^{-1/m}(\xi) & \text{if } \det M(\xi) \neq 0, \\ \infty & \text{if } \det M(\xi) = 0. \end{cases}$$

One of the main reasons for the definition with the log is that the determinant is sometimes so small that it produces some computational problems. The log scale may help to solve this problem. On the other hand, the gradient is friendlier than in the second case. And, finally, this form helps to prove convexity of the criterion function through arguments of log-convex functions, although both are convex.

Remark 2.2 The determinant of a matrix is not concave, but the determinant of the inverse is convex. This is a fact that is not always stressed in the OED literature and sometimes it is even denied. There are some nontrivial proofs that the logarithm of the determinant of a matrix is concave (see, e.g., Pázman, 1986, Proposition IV.2). Then changing the sign of this function there is the logarithm of the determinant of the inverse matrix, which is then convex. This is what typically is call log-convexity, in this case of the determinant of the inverse of a matrix. A well-known result states that if a function is log-convex then it is convex. Therefore, the determinant of the inverse of a matrix should be convex. In the same way $\det M^{-1/m}$ must be convex.

These are some properties:

1. Φ_D is continuous and convex on $\mathcal{M}$, and strictly convex on $\mathcal{M}_+$ (nonsingular information matrices).
2. It is differentiable on $\mathcal{M}_+$,

$$\nabla(-\log \det M) = -M^{-1},$$

$$\nabla(\det M^{-1/m}) = \frac{1}{m} M^{-1} \det M^{-1/m}.$$

3. This criterion minimizes the volume of the confidence ellipsoid of the parameters,

$$(\hat{\theta} - \theta)^T (X^T X)^{-1} (\hat{\theta} - \theta) \leq m F_{m,n-m,\gamma} S_R^2 \equiv c^2.$$

It is well-known that the volume of the ellipsoid is $c^m V_m [\det M^{-1}(\xi)]^{1/2}$, where V_m is the volume of the m-dimensional sphere.

Some explicit formulae for the determinant of an FIM may help in practice. There is an especial but usual case when the number of design points is equal to the number of parameters, $k = m$, then let

$$m_{ij} = \sum_{r=1}^{m} f_i(x_r) f_j(x_r) \xi(x_r).$$

Let $A = \{a_{ir}\}$ and $B = \{b_{jr}\}$, where $a_{ir} = f_i(x_r)\xi(x_r)$ and $b_{jr} = f_j(x_r)$, then

$$\det M(\xi) = \det A \det B = \prod_{r=1}^{m} \xi(x_r) \det \left[\{f_i(x_j)\}\right]^2.$$

Since in this formula weights and model are separated in different factors, a consequence is that *any D-optimal design with m points in its support has equal weights*. This helps very much in the general computation of D-optimal designs.

There is also an expression for the general case, $k \geq m$ (Pázman, 1986, Proposition V.8),

$$
\begin{aligned}
\det M(\xi) &= \det \left[\left\{ \sum_{r=1}^{k} f_i(x_r) f_j(x_r) \xi(x_r) \right\}_{ij} \right] \\
&= \sum_{r_1 < \cdots < r_m \leq k} \det[\{f_i(x_{r_j}) f_j(x_{r_j}) \xi(x_{r_j})\}_{ij}] \\
&= \sum_{r_1 < \cdots < r_m \leq k} \prod_{j=1}^{m} \xi(x_{r_j}) \det \left[\{f_i(x_{r_j})\}_{ij} \right]^2
\end{aligned}
$$

Last inequality comes from the first case.

2.4.4 G-optimality

D-optimality focuses mainly on the estimation of the parameters of the model. If the aim is prediction, a possible criterion is G-optimality. Its origin goes as far as the starting point of Optimal Design of Experiments with a pioneering long paper by Smith (1918). Then (Kiefer & Wolfowitz, 1960) put the name of G-optimality (from Generalized variance of the predictions). The criterion is defined as follows:

$$
\Phi_G[M(\xi)] = \begin{cases} \max_{x \in \mathcal{X}} f^T(x) M^{-1}(\xi) f(x) & \text{if } \det M(\xi) \neq 0, \\ \infty & \text{if } \det M(\xi) = 0, \end{cases}
$$

where $d(x, \xi) = f^T(x) M^{-1}(\xi) f(x)$ is proportional to the variance of the prediction $\hat{y}(x)$.

The criterion function Φ_G is continuous and convex on $\mathcal{M}$. In general, this criterion is not differentiable since there is no guarantee that the maximum of differentiable functions is differentiable. Although D- and G-optimality have two very different aims in both mathematical and statistical meaning, Kiefer and Wolfowitz (1960) proved they produced the same optimal designs. A priori it might be expected that a design could be quite good for estimation and rather bad for prediction, but this is not the case. This is at least for the best designs for both purposes.

2.4.5 A-optimality

Another meaningful criterion is the average of the variances, that is, the trace of the inverse of the FIM,

$$\Phi_A[M(\xi)] = \begin{cases} \text{tr}M^{-1}(\xi) \propto \sum_{i=1}^m \text{var}(\hat{\theta}_i) & \text{if } \det M(\xi) \neq 0 \\ \infty & \text{if } \det M(\xi) = 0, \end{cases}$$

The second equality is a consequence of

$$\text{var}\hat{\theta}_i \propto u_i^t M^{-1}(\xi) u_i$$

if the parameters are estimable (nonsingular matrix), where the vectors $u_1, \ldots, u_m$ form the canonical basis.

The criterion Φ_A is continuous and convex on $\mathcal{M}$ and strictly convex on $\mathcal{M}_+$. It is also differentiable on $\mathcal{M}_+$ and the gradient is

$$\nabla(\text{tr}M^{-1}(\xi)) = -M^{-2}(\xi).$$

Given m different points $x_1, x_2, \ldots, x_m$, the best weights according to A-optimality are (Pukelsheim & Torsney, 1991),

$$p_i^\star = \frac{\sqrt{m_{ii}}}{\sum_{j=1}^m \sqrt{m_{jj}}}, \quad j = 1, \ldots, m,$$

where $(XX^T)^{-1} = \{m_{ij}\}_{ij}$ and X is the design matrix for these points without weights. This is a very useful result to compute A-optimal designs when the number of design points is equal to the number of parameters.

Remark 2.3

1. This criterion is not appropriate when the variances of the estimators of the parameters are of different magnitudes; for instance, when the regressors are of different scale, then the criterion pays too much attention to large-scale parameters and almost nothing to a small-scale parameter. For instance, assume a model with several variables where one is the weight. Using weights measured in grams or kilograms may take to very different designs, although the situation is exactly the same. Thus, some normalization is needed here (Dette, 1997; López-Fidalgo et al., 2007a).
2. We have seen that the gradient for the determinant and the trace is minus the inverse of the information matrix and its square, respectively. These are the extremal symmetric functions in the decomposition of the characteristic polynomial of the matrix. Rodríguez-Díaz and López-Fidalgo (2003) considered the intermediate symmetric functions producing interesting criterion functions in the middle. They proved the convexity and differentiability of those criteria and

provided the gradient for all of them. They are specially interesting for multiple comparisons.

2.4.6 L-optimality

Atwood (1976) provided a class of "linear criteria" aiming to optimize the estimation of linear combinations of the parameters, which is rather practical in some situations. Let H be a $m \times l$ matrix with maximum rank $l \leq m$ defining l linear combinations of the parameters. The criterion is defined as

$$\Phi_L[M(\xi)] = \begin{cases} \text{tr} H^T M^-(\xi) H & \text{if } \text{Img}(H) \subset \text{Img}[M(\xi)], \\ \infty & \text{otherwise,} \end{cases}$$

where Img(·) stands for the image of the linear function generated by a matrix (see A).

The function Φ_L is continuous and convex on $\mathcal{M}$. It is differentiable at the designs such that if all the combinations are identifiable, with gradient

$$\nabla[\text{tr} H^T M^{-1}(\xi) H] = -M^{-1}(\xi) H H^T M^{-1}(\xi).$$

Given m different points $x_1, x_2, \ldots, x_m$, Pukelsheim and Torsney (1991) provided a method to compute the best weights according to L-optimality. Sometimes this criterion is defined for as $\text{tr} W M^-(\xi)$, where $W = H H^T$ is nonnegative definite. Both definitions are equivalent and they will be used indistinctly along the book.

2.4.7 E-optimality

One of the possible problems with D-optimality is that the volume of the confidence ellipsoid can be minimum, while one of the axes is quite large. Since the length of the axes is proportional to the square root of the eigenvalues of the inverse of the FIM, then minimizing the maximum of the eigenvalues looks directly for the problem mentioned at the beginning. This is a version of the criterion of E-optimality aiming this,

$$\Phi_E[M(\xi)] = \sup \left\{ \text{var} \hat{\theta}^T c \, : \, ||c|| = 1 \right\}, \; \xi \in \Xi.$$

This is another minimax criterion and $\Phi_E[M(\xi)] = \infty$ if and only if there exists a linear combination $\theta^T c$ nonestimable for ξ, that is, if $M(\xi)$ is singular.

This definition means that this criterion minimizes the test power of the usual F-test for testing whether a certain linear combination of the parameters is zero.

If $M(\xi)$ is nonsingular, let $\lambda_1, \ldots, \lambda_m$ be the eigenvalues, let λ_ξ be the minimum eigenvalue, and let $u_1, \ldots, u_m$ be the eigenvectors. Then,

$$M^{-1}(\xi)u_i = \lambda_i^{-1}u_i,\ i = 1, 2, \ldots, m$$

and

$$\sup\left\{c^T M^{-1}(\xi)c : \| c \| = 1\right\} \geq u_i^t M^{-1}(\xi)u_i = \lambda_i^{-1},\ i = 1, 2, \ldots, m.$$

For each vector c with $\| c \| = 1$ such that $c = \sum_{i=1}^m a_i u_i$, with $\sum_i a_i^2 = 1$,

$$c^T M^{-1}(\xi)c = \sum_{i,j} a_i u_i^t M^{-1}(\xi)u_j a_j \leq \lambda_\xi^{-1},$$

taking into account that $u_i^t M^{-1}(\xi)u_j = 0,\ i \neq j$.

Therefore,

$$\Phi_E[M(\xi)] = \begin{cases} \lambda_\xi^{-1} & \text{if } \det M(\xi) \neq 0, \\ \infty & \text{if } \det M(\xi) = 0. \end{cases}$$

Φ_E is continuous and convex on $\mathcal{M}$.

2.4.8 MV-optimality

Another meaningful criterion is to minimize the largest of the variances of the estimators of the parameters, that is, the maximum of the diagonal of the inverse of the FIM,

$$\Phi_{MV}[M(\xi)] = \begin{cases} \max_i \operatorname{var}\hat{\theta}_i & \text{if } \det M(\xi) \neq 0, \\ \infty & \text{if } \det M(\xi) = 0. \end{cases}$$

That is,

$$\Phi_{MV}[M(\xi)] = \begin{cases} \max_i \left\{M^{-1}(\xi)\right\}_{ii} & \text{if } \det M(\xi) \neq 0, \\ \infty & \text{if } \det M(\xi) = 0. \end{cases}$$

Remark 2.4 Again this criterion is not appropriate when the variances of the parameters are of different magnitudes. Then it needs some normalization (Dette, 1997; López-Fidalgo et al., 2007a).

2.4.9 I-optimality

This criterion is an alternative to G-optimality for prediction. Instead of optimizing the worst prediction within the design space, I-optimality will optimize the mean value of the variances of the predictions according to a probability measure, μ, on a particular set S of interest for predictions. This set would typically be the design space, but it can be part of it or some set with points further the design space. The criterion function is defined by

$$\Phi_I[M(\xi)] = \begin{cases} \int_S f^T(x)M^{-1}(\xi)f(x)\mu(dx) & \text{if } \det M(\xi) \neq 0, \\ \infty & \text{if } \det M(\xi) = 0. \end{cases}$$

This criterion is equivalent to L-optimality for $W = \int_S f(x)f^T(x)\mu(dx)$, since

$$\int_S f^T(x)M^{-1}(\xi)f(x)\mu(dx) = \text{tr}\left[\int_S f(x)f^T(x)\mu(dx)M^{-1}(\xi)\right] = \text{tr}[WM^{-1}(\xi)].$$

2.4.10 Φ_p-optimality

This criteria family was first introduced by Kiefer (1974) trying to summarize some of the already "invented" criteria. The criterion is defined for any $m \times \nu$ ($\nu \leq m$) matrix H and for $p > 0$,

$$\Phi_p[M(\xi)] = \begin{cases} \left\{\frac{1}{\nu}\text{tr}[H^T M^{-1}(\xi)H]^p\right\}^{1/p} & \text{if } \text{Img}(H) \subset \text{Img}(M(\xi)) \text{ and } \det M(\xi) \neq 0, \\ \infty & \text{otherwise,} \end{cases}$$

where Img(·) stands for the image of the linear function generated by a matrix (see A).

The criterion is convex and for nonsingular designs it is differentiable with gradient

$$\nabla\{\Phi_p[M(\xi)]\} = -\frac{1}{p\nu^{1/p}}\left\{\text{tr}[H^T M^{-}(\xi)H]^p\right\}^{1/p-1}\sum_{h=0}^{p-1}[M^{h-p}(\xi)(HH^T)^p M^{-h-1}(\xi).$$

For $p = 1$ we have L-optimality, when $p \to 0$ the criterion becomes D-optimality and finally E-optimality when $p \to \infty$.

2.4.11 D_s-optimality

This criterion focuses on some of the parameters, say $s < m$, according to the determinant criterion. Thus, it will minimize the determinant of the covariance matrix of the estimators of the parameters of interest. Let us assume without loss of generality these s parameters are the first ones and denote

$$M(\xi) = \begin{pmatrix} [M(\xi)]_{11} & [M(\xi)]_{12} \\ [M(\xi)]_{21} & [M(\xi)]_{22} \end{pmatrix},$$

$$M^{-}(\xi) = \begin{pmatrix} [M^{-}(\xi)]_{11} & [M^{-}(\xi)]_{12} \\ [M^{-}(\xi)]_{21} & [M^{-}(\xi)]_{22} \end{pmatrix},$$

where $-$ stands for a pseudo-inverse matrix and $[M(\xi)]_{11}$, $[M^{-}(\xi)]_{11}$ are block matrices of order s corresponding to the parameters of interest. The design criterion is then defined as

$$\Phi_{D_s}[M(\xi)] = \begin{cases} \{\det[M^{-}(\xi)]_{11}\}^{1/s} & \text{if } u_i \in \text{Img}M(\xi),\ i = 1, \ldots, s, \\ \infty & \text{otherwise,} \end{cases}$$

where $u_1, \ldots, u_m$ is the canonical basis.

If $M(\xi)$ is singular $M^{-}(\xi)$ is not unique, but the condition $u_i \in \text{Img}M(\xi)$, $i = 1, \ldots, s$ implies the block matrix $[M^{-}(\xi)]_{11}$ is unique (see Appendix A) and therefore the definition is coherent.

If $M(\xi)$ is nonsingular, using formulas for the inverse and the determinant of a matrix defined by blocks (see Appendix A), the criterion has a friendly form,

$$\Phi_{D_s}[M(\xi)] = \left\{ \frac{\det[M(\xi)]_{22}}{\det[M(\xi)]} \right\}^{1/s}.$$

2.4.12 c-optimality

This is another local criterion focused on minimizing the variance of the estimator of $c^T\theta$, a linear combination of the parameters defined by the vector $c^T = (c_1, \ldots, c_m)$,

$$\Phi_c[M(\xi)] = \begin{cases} c^T M^{-}(\xi) c & \text{if } c \in \text{Img}M(\xi), \\ \infty. & \text{otherwise.} \end{cases}$$

If $M(\xi)$ is singular $M^{-}(\xi)$ is not unique, but the condition $c \in \text{Img}M(\xi)$ implies $c^T M^{-}(\xi) c$ is unique and therefore the definition is coherent.

Actually, this criterion is D$_1$-optimality when $s = 1$ and $c^T = (1, 0, \ldots, 0)$, applicable to any of the parameters. Elfving (1952) provided an elegant procedure to compute graphically c-optimal designs. This is being considered in the next section.

Given m different points $x_1, x_2, \ldots, x_m$ the best weights according to c-optimality are (Pukelsheim & Torsney, 1991),

$$p_i^\star = \frac{\sqrt{v_i}}{\sum_{j=1}^{m} \sqrt{v_j}}, \quad j = 1, \ldots, m,$$

where $v = (XX^T)^{-1}Xc$ and X is the design matrix for these points without weights.

Example 2.5 Revisiting Example 2.4, let us compare the three rounded-off designs to see which one is better according to different criteria. For that we used the FIM coming from the probability measure defined by the exact designs; thus, they may be compared with the approximate design. These are the designs to be compared,

$$\xi = \left\{ \begin{matrix} 0 & 0.5 & 1 \\ 0.2 & 0.4 & 0.4 \end{matrix} \right\}, \quad \xi_{12}^\star = \left\{ \begin{matrix} 0 & 0.5 & 1 \\ 2/12 & 5/12 & 5/12 \end{matrix} \right\}$$

$$\xi_{12}^{\star\star} = \left\{ \begin{matrix} 0 & 0.5 & 1 \\ 3/12 & 4/12 & 5/12 \end{matrix} \right\}, \quad \xi_{12}^{\star\star\star} = \left\{ \begin{matrix} 0 & 0.5 & 1 \\ 3/12 & 5/12 & 4/12 \end{matrix} \right\}.$$

Table 2.1 shows the values of different criterion functions for the four designs. Second row displays the determinants of the FIMs. Design $\xi_{12}^{\star\star}$ has the greater value among all, including the original one. For the other criteria it is rather similar. For A-optimality the last two rounded-off designs improve the original design. In particular, $\xi_{12}^{\star\star}$ is the best one, although this one does not come from the usual rounding-off procedure. For E-optimality the maximum eigenvalues are displayed and again $\xi_{12}^{\star\star}$ is the best. If there is special interest in estimating optimally the slope, then we have c-optimality for $c^T = (0, 1)$ and the last row of the table shows again that the best design is $\xi_{12}^{\star\star}$. This makes much sense since the optimal designs for each criterion are nearer this one. Later we will compare previous designs with the optimal design for each criterion using the right efficiency and some bounds provided after giving the equivalence theorem.

Table 2.1 Values of different criterion functions for the four designs. For c-optimality the vector considered is $c^T = (0, 1)$. Second row displays the determinants of the FIMs

Design	ξ	$\xi_{12}^\star$	$\xi_{12}^{\star\star}$	$\xi_{12}^{\star\star\star}$
Determinant	0.140	0.130	0.160	0.144
Trace	10.714	11.680	9.391	9.976
Largest eigenvalue	10.00	10.98	8.67	9.22
Variance for c	7.143	7.680	6.261	6.940

2.5 Elfving Graphical Procedure for c-Optimality

Elfving (1952) gave an elegant procedure to compute c-optimal designs graphically. This procedure is mainly used for two-parameter models. Graphical visualization is rather tedious for three parameters and impossible for more than three. López-Fidalgo and Rodríguez-Díaz (2004) gave a procedure based on this to find c-optimal designs for more than two parameters. Later on Harman and Jurik (2008); Harman and Stulajter (2010), and Bartroff (2011) have improved this procedure.

Let

$$y = f_1(x)\theta_1 + \cdots + f_m(x)\theta_m + \varepsilon, \sigma^2(x) = \sigma^2, x \in \chi$$

be a linear model.

Let ξ_n be an exact design $x_1, \ldots, x_k$ with weights $p_i = n_i/n$ (n_i observations at each x_i). Thus, this design determines k points in the Euclidean space $\mathbb{R}^m$,

$$f^T(x_1) = (f_1(x_1), \ldots, f_m(x_1)), \ldots, f^T(x_k) = (f_1(x_k), \ldots, f_m(x_k)).$$

The means of observations at x_i give

$$\bar{y}_i = f_1(x_i)\theta_1 + \cdots + f_m(x_i)\theta_m + \bar{\varepsilon}_i,$$

where $\text{var}(\bar{y}_i) = \sigma^2/n_i$.

The interest is in estimating a linear combination of the parameters, say $c^T\theta$ with $c^T = (c_1, \ldots, c_m)$. Let us assume an estimator, linear on the responses,

$$\widehat{c^T\theta} = \sum_{i=1}^{k} a_i \bar{y}_i.$$

It is unbiased if

$$\text{E}(\widehat{c^T\theta}) = \sum_{i=1}^{k} a_i[f_1(x_i)\theta_1 + \cdots + f_m(x_i)\theta_m] = c_1\theta_1 \cdots + c_m\theta_m,$$

that is,

$$\sum_{i=1}^{k} a_i f(x_i) = c.$$

The variance must be minimal,

$$\mathrm{var}(\widehat{c^T\theta}) = \mathrm{var}\left(\sum_{i=1}^k a_i \bar{y}_i\right) = \sum_{i=1}^k a_i^2 \mathrm{var}\,(\bar{y}_i) = \frac{\sigma^2}{n}\sum_{i=1}^k a_i^2 \frac{n}{n_i}$$

$$= \frac{\sigma^2}{n}\sum_{i=1}^k \frac{a_i^2}{\xi_n(x_i)}.$$

For fixed values of a_i, $i = 1, \ldots, k$, and exchanging the exact design here, $\xi_n(x_i)$ for any design ξ with this support, the minimal variance is reached for the weights $\xi_a(x_i) = |a_i|/\sum_{i=1}^k |a_i| = |a_i|/||a||_1$, where $||a||_1$ is the ℓ^1 norm of vector $a^T = (a_1, \ldots, a_k)$. This can be proved with the Lagrange multipliers using the constraint $1 = \sum_{i=1}^k \xi(x_i)$. Then,

$$\frac{n}{\sigma^2}\mathrm{var}(\widehat{c^T\theta}) = \sum_{i=1}^k \frac{a_i^2}{\xi_a(x_i)} = \sum_{i=1}^k \frac{a_i^2||a||_1}{|a_i|} = ||a||_1 \sum_{i=1}^k |a_i| = ||a||_1^2.$$

The unbiased condition is now transformed to

$$c = \sum_{i=1}^k a_i f(x_i) = ||a||_1 \sum_{i=1}^k \xi_a(x_i)\ \mathrm{sgn}(a_i) f(x_i) = ||a||_1 c_a$$

for some vector c_a proportional to c. Values $a_1, \ldots, a_k$ should minimize $||a||_1^2$ subject to this condition, where c_a must be a convex combination of points of $f(\chi) \cup -f(\chi)$.

The weights $\xi_a(x_i)$, $i = 1, \ldots, k$ are nonnegative and sum up to one. Thus, the extreme is in the boundary of the convex hull of $f(\chi) \cup -f(\chi) = \{\pm f(x_1), \ldots, \pm f(x_k)\}$. We will refer to this as the *Elfving set*. Figure 2.1 shows this situation in a simple example with just three points in the design support. The minimal variance is reached at $c_a = \sum_{i=1}^k \xi_a(x_i)\mathrm{sgn}(a_i) f(x_i)$, defined by the

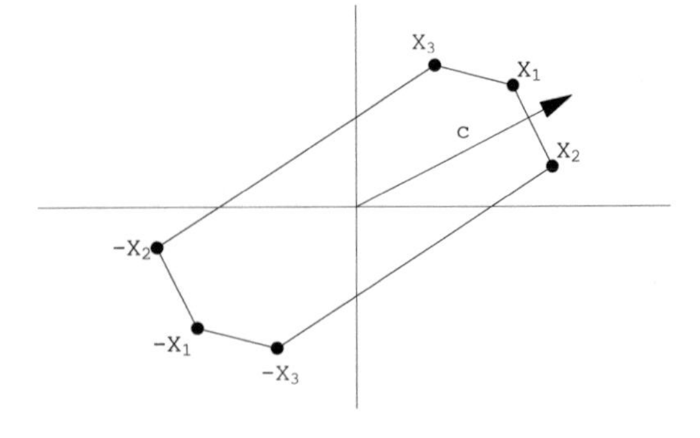

Fig. 2.1 Convex hull of $f(\chi) \cup -f(\chi)$ for just three points in the design space

intersection between the straight line defined by c and the boundary of the convex hull of $f(\chi) \cup -f(\chi)$. Moreover, the variance is proportional to $||a||_1 = \frac{||c||_2}{||c_a||_2}$.

This method is quite visual for two parameters and still usable for some models with three parameters. For higher dimension, López-Fidalgo and Rodríguez-Díaz (2004) gave a procedure based on these results and (Harman and Stulajter, 2010; Bartroff, 2011) improved it.

Remark 2.5 Frequently there is interest in estimating the maximum of the model of the mean, the point where this maximum is reached or the area under the curve (AUC), to mention a few possibilities. Very often this function is nonlinear on the parameters. Thus, let $g(\theta)$ be a differentiable function of the parameters. If $\hat{\theta}$ are the MLEs of the parameters, the estimator $g(\hat{\theta})$ has an asymptotic variance

$$\frac{\partial g(\theta)}{\partial \theta^T} M^{-1}(\xi) \frac{\partial g(\theta)}{\partial \theta}.$$

Then for some nominal values of the parameters, θ_0, the optimal design can be approximated by the c-optimal design for $c = \left(\frac{\partial g(\theta)}{\partial \theta}\right)_{\theta=\theta_0}$.

2.5.1 *Elfving's Procedure in Practice*

Let a linear model with mean of the observations $\theta_1 f_1(t) + \theta_2 f_2(t)$. As an abuse of notation in what follows x and y will denote the axes where the Elfving set is represented as it is usual in geometry. For the explanatory variable t is used in this section, while the response is not needed here.

1. Plot the curve $x(t) = f_1(t),\ y(t) = f_2(t), t \in \chi$ and its symmetric through the origin.
2. Plot the convex hull of both curves. In a continuous space this will frequently be a matter of drawing tangent straight lines.
3. Plot the line through the origin defined by vector c until the boundary if necessary.
4. The optimal design is defined by the boundary point intersecting the straight line defined by c.

Figures 2.2 and 2.3 show an example for $f_1(x) = e^{-x},\ f_2(x) = xe^{-x},\ \chi = [0, 3]$. Figure 2.2 shows that for a vector $c^T = (1, 0.5)$, the c-optimal design has just one point in its support,

$$\left\{ \begin{matrix} z \\ 1 \end{matrix} \right\},$$

while for $c^T = (-0.7, 0.4)$ the c-optimal design needs two points (Fig. 2.2).

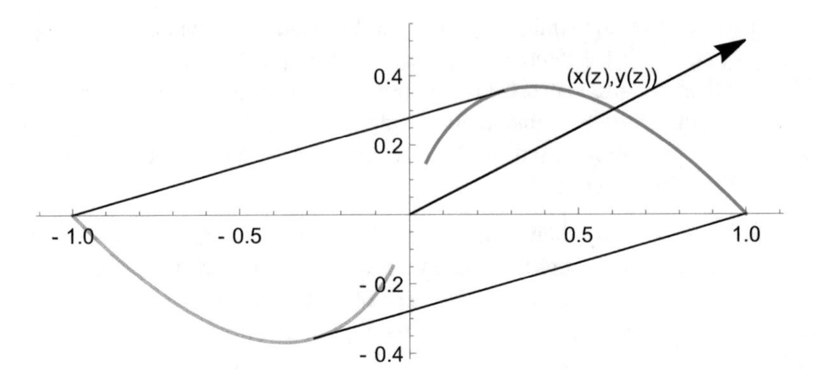

Fig. 2.2 Elfving plot for a one-point c-optimal design

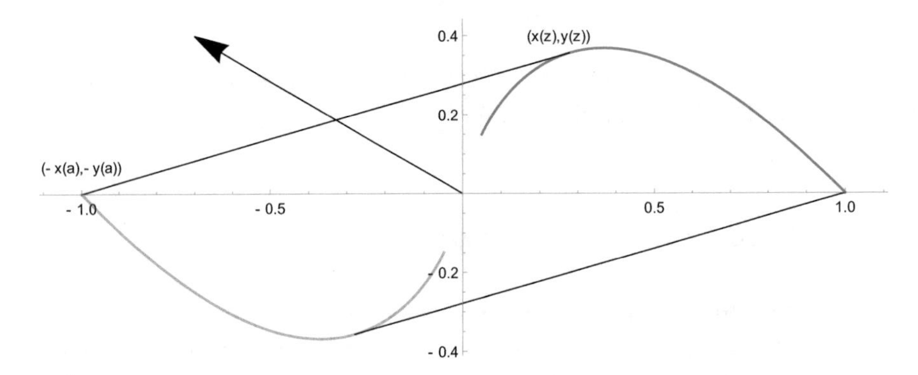

Fig. 2.3 Elfving plot for a two-point design

Figure 2.3 shows an example for a two-point c-optimal design,

$$\left\{ \begin{matrix} a & z \\ 1 - p^{\star} & p^{\star} \end{matrix} \right\}$$

2.5.2 *Computing Tangential Points*

The straight line between a tangential point from $-f(\chi)$ and an extreme point from $f(\chi)$ (Figs. 2.2 and 2.3), say $(x(a), y(a))$, can be computed as the solution of the equation

$$\frac{x(a) + x(t)}{x'(t)} = \frac{y(a) + y(t)}{y'(t)}.$$

The straight line between two tangential points, one from $f(\chi)$ and one from $-f(\chi)$, is computed as a solution of the two-equation system,

$$\frac{x(t)+x(s)}{x'(s)} = \frac{y(t)+y(s)}{y'(s)},$$

$$\frac{x'(t)}{x'(s)} = \frac{y'(t)}{y'(s)}.$$

A simple example will illustrate this.

Example 2.6 Let the model be

$$E[y] = \theta^T f(x) = \theta_1 x + \theta_2 x^2, \sigma^2(x) = 1,\ x \in \chi = [0, 1].$$

Then the curve $x(t) = t,\ y(t) = t^2, t \in [0, 1]$ is shown in Fig. 2.4 (left) and the symmetric plot through the origin is in Fig. 2.4 (right).

Figure 2.5 shows the convex hull defined by one tangential point. This actually means there are two types of c-optimal designs in two dimensions. They can be two-point designs, always supported at 0.4142 and 1, or one-point designs between these two points.

The tangential point, z, is computed solving the equation

$$\frac{x(z)-x_0}{x'(z)} = \frac{y(z)-y_0}{y'(z)},$$

that is,

$$\frac{z+1}{1} = \frac{z^2+1}{2z},\ z = \sqrt{2}-1.$$

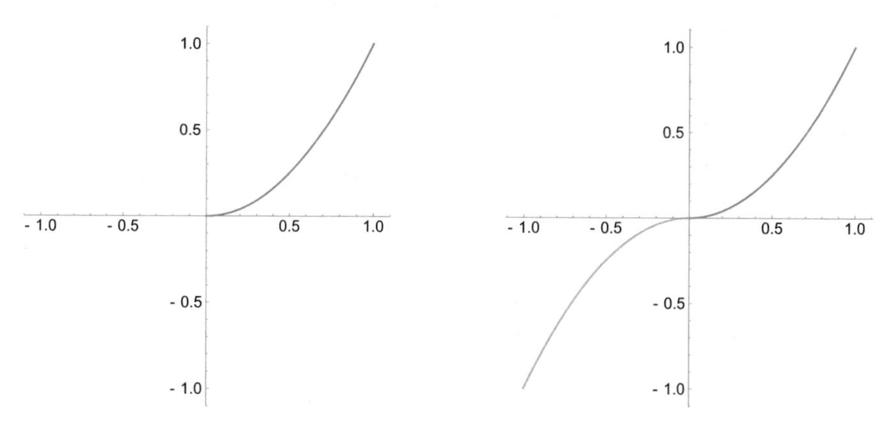

Fig. 2.4 Elfving locus

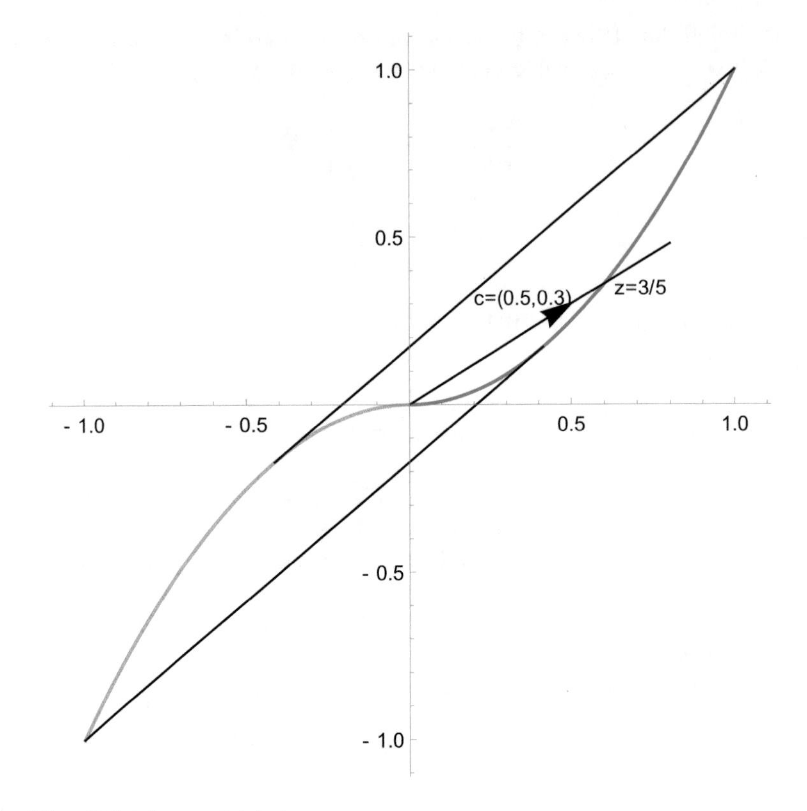

Fig. 2.5 c-Optimal one-point design

Let us consider first the vector $c = (0.5, 0.3)$. Figure 2.5 shows this vector cuts the curve giving a one-point design,

$$(0.5\lambda)^2 = 0.3\lambda, \; t = 3/5$$

$$\xi_c^\star = \begin{Bmatrix} 3/5 \\ 1 \end{Bmatrix}$$

Let $c = (0.5, 1)$ be another vector. Figure 2.6 shows the c-optimal is now a two-point design.

The cutting point is computed as follows:

$$\begin{cases} y = 2x, \\ \frac{x-1}{z+1} = \frac{y-1}{z^2+1}, \end{cases}$$

$$x = \frac{1}{4}\left(2 - \sqrt{2}\right) = 0.15, \; y = 0.30,$$

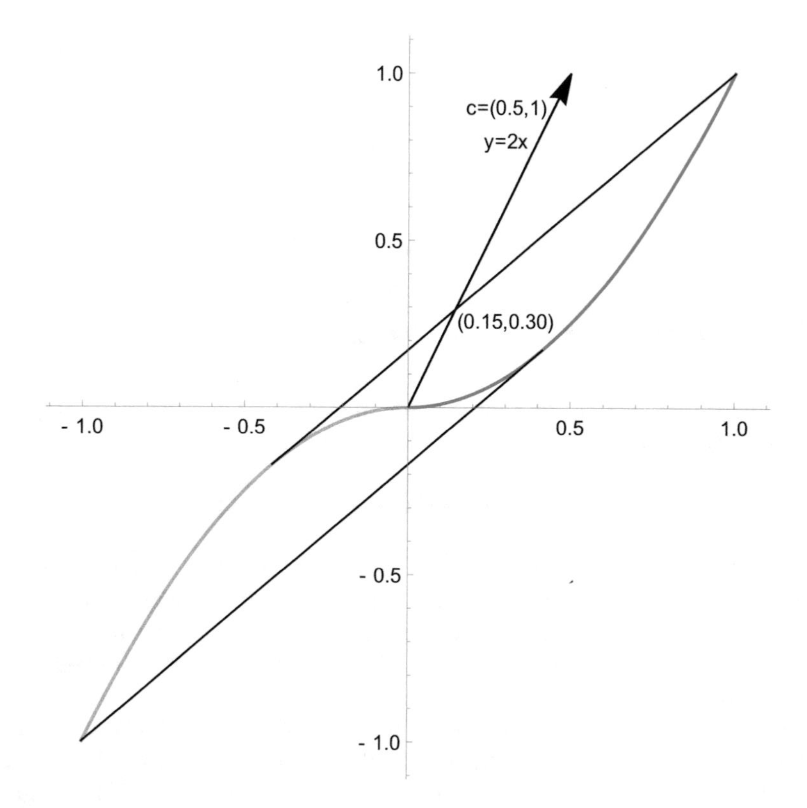

Fig. 2.6 c-Optimal two-point design

and the weights come from the convex combination

$$(0.15, 0.30) = (1 - p)(-z, -z^2) + p(1, 1),\ p = \frac{1}{4}\left(3 - \sqrt{2}\right) = 0.30.$$

Therefore

$$\xi_c^\star = \left\{ \begin{array}{cc} \sqrt{2} - 1 & 1 \\ \frac{1}{4}\left(1 + \sqrt{2}\right) & \frac{1}{4}\left(3 - \sqrt{2}\right) \end{array} \right\}$$

is the c-optimal design.

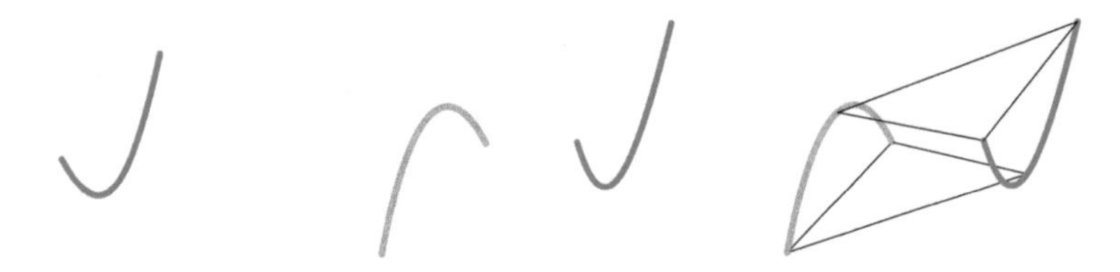

Fig. 2.7 Three-dimensional Elfving set for the quadratic model

2.5.3 Procedure for Three or More Parameters

Figure 2.7 shows the graphical construction of the convex hull of the Elfving locus for a quadratic model,

$$y = \theta_1 + \theta_2 t + \theta_3 t^2 + \varepsilon, t \in [-1, 1].$$

Although this is a very simple case with a planar curve, it can be seen the difficulty of using directly this method. The two triangles correspond to three-point designs, while the rest are two-point designs, except the vectors touching the curves, which they are one-point optimal designs. Other cases are much more complex to solve using these ideas.

Frequently, the interest is not in estimating all the parameters of the model but some linear combination. A particular case is when there is special interest in estimating just one parameter. The Elfving's method (Elfving, 1952) is a graph procedure for calculating c-optimal designs. Although the method can be applied to any number of parameters, it is not used directly for more than two parameters. López-Fidalgo and Rodríguez-Díaz (2004) proposed a computational procedure for finding c-optimal designs using Elfving's method for more than two dimensions.

Figure 2.8 shows example with three parameters, where the Elfving set, convex hull of $f(\chi) \cup -f(\chi)$, is rather complex to visualize the optimal designs. López-Fidalgo and Rodríguez-Díaz (2004)'s procedure can be applied here in a friendly way.

The idea is rather simple although the formal way of describing it needs unpleasant notation. Assuming the Elfving set all it is needed is to find the intersection of the line defined by vector c and the boundary of the Elfving set. The two possible points are just symmetric and produce the same design. This point has to be a convex combination of several points of the set $f(\chi) \cup -f(\chi)$. Those points will be the support points of the c-optimal design and the coefficients of the convex combination will be the weights of the design. Computing this point for two parameters is rather simple, but for more parameters, even just three, it is not affordable or too complex.

López-Fidalgo and Rodríguez-Díaz (2004)'s procedure is as follows. Consider any of the non-null components of c, say the first one without loss of generality. Let a general point satisfying the conditions of the Elfving set, that is, a convex

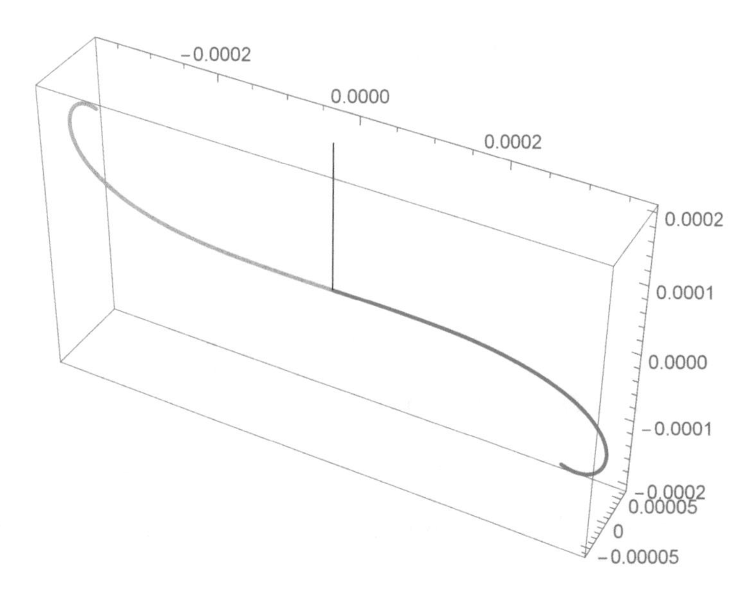

Fig. 2.8 Elfving set (properly scaled)

combination of no more than m points of $f(\chi) \cup -f(\chi)$. The first component can be considered as the objective function to be maximize (or minimize). This generic point depends actually on m different points and $m - 1$ coefficients. Now they must satisfy that they are in the straight line defined by c, so the point must be proportional to c, say δc, for some scalar δ. This gives m linear (in the coefficients) equations with the extra δ. All the coefficients can be worked out easily.

Thus, the objective function is any of the components of the point such that $c_i \neq 0$, which depends just on the m points of the design. This is a standard optimization problem with a number of algorithms and software available for computing the optimal. This procedure will be shown in detail with the example considered in this work.

To show the general idea in an easier way we will restrict to three dimensions with $c^T = (0, 0, 1)$; that is, the interest is in estimating the third parameter of the model.

The c-optimal design will be of the form

$$\xi = \left\{ \begin{matrix} t & s & u \\ 1 - \lambda - \delta & \lambda & \delta \end{matrix} \right\},$$

corresponding to a point on the boundary of the Elfving set as well as it remains on the line defined by $c = (0, 0, 1)$. Some weights can be zero, leading to two- or one-point designs. Thus, all the possible cases are considered here. A point in the Elfving set has to be a convex combination of, at least, three points of $f(\chi) \cup -f(\chi)$. Apart from symmetric situations there are two possibilities. The three points come from

$f(\chi)$ (symmetrically from $-f(\chi)$), that is,

$$(x, y, z)^T = (1 - \lambda - \delta) f(t) + \lambda f(s) + \delta f(u)$$

or two come from $f(\chi)$ and one from $-f(\chi)$ (symmetrically two come from $-f(\chi)$ and one from $f(\chi)$), that is,

$$(x, y, z)^T = (1 - \lambda - \delta) f(t) + \lambda f(s) - \delta f(u).$$

For instance, the example in Fig. 2.8 suggests the point will be of the second kind with tree support points. At the same time they must be on the line defined by $c^T = (0, 0, 1)$. Thus, for the second case,

$$(1 - \lambda - \delta) f(t) + \lambda f(s) - \delta f(u) = \rho(0, 0, 1)^T.$$

The equations coming from the two first components give the values of λ and δ in function on the three points

$$\begin{aligned} (1 - \lambda - \delta) f_1(t) + \lambda f_1(s) - \delta f_1(u) &= 0, \\ (1 - \lambda - \delta) f_2(t) + \lambda f_2(s) - \delta f_2(u) &= 0, \end{aligned} \tag{2.3}$$

that is, $\lambda(t, s, u)$ and $\delta(t, s, u)$. Plugging them into the third component, the function

$$z(t, s, u) = [1 - \lambda(t, s, u) - \delta(t, s, u)] f_3(t) + \lambda(t, s, u) f_3(s) - \delta(t, s, u) f_3(u) \tag{2.4}$$

has to be maximized subject to $t, s, u \in \chi$. This is a very typical optimization problem, which may be solved using any mathematical software. Once the optimal points, $t^\star$, $s^\star$, and $u^\star$, are computed, the weights are them obtained from the solutions of Eqs. (2.3).

Example 2.7 For illustrating this procedure the quadratic model mentioned at the beginning of this section is being considered,

$$f^T(x) = (1, x, x^2),\ x \in [-1, 1],\ c^T = (0, 0, 1).$$

Figure 2.7 shows the line defined by c crosses the boundary of the convex hull at some interior point of the triangle. Therefore, it is a convex combination of the two extremes and some interior point. Thus, the point is of the second kind considered above. Solving the Eqs. (2.3),

$$(1-\lambda-\delta)+\lambda-\delta=0,$$
$$(1-\lambda-\delta)t+\lambda s-\delta u=0,$$

then

$$\lambda=\frac{t-u}{2(t-s)},\ \delta=1/2.$$

Plugging then into (2.4),

$$z(t,s,u)=\frac{1}{2}(s-u)(u-t),$$

and the maximum of this function is reached at $s=-1,\ u=0,\ t=1$. Then their weights can be computed plugging then into the solutions given for the coefficients, $\lambda=1/4$ and $\delta=1/2$, and the design is

$$\xi_c^\star=\begin{Bmatrix} -1 & 0 & 1 \\ 1/4 & 1/2 & 1/4 \end{Bmatrix}.$$

2.6 The Equivalence Theorem

This mathematical result, valid just for approximate designs, provides a powerful tool for the optimal design theory and practice. The first version of the theorem established an equivalence between D- and G-optimality (Kiefer & Wolfowitz, 1960). Then (Whittle, 1973) used the idea to extend the theorem to convex criteria. This version provides a way of checking whether a particular design is optimal or not. From this theorem efficiency bounds can be given and sequential algorithms to compute optimal designs can be built. In this section the more general definition of criterion function will be used. Thus, all the results will be valid for both definitions.

A definition of the *directional derivative* of Φ at ζ in the direction of ζ' is needed here,

$$\partial\Phi(\zeta,\zeta')=\lim_{\epsilon\to 0^+}\frac{\Phi[(1-\epsilon)\zeta+\epsilon\zeta']-\Phi(\zeta)}{\epsilon}.$$

This is actually the so-called directional derivative of Gâteaux and it coincides with the usual directional derivative of Φ at ζ in the direction of $\zeta'-\zeta$. This definition is convenient here since the set of the information matrices is convex and therefore the matrix $(1-\epsilon)M+\epsilon N$ is still an information matrix.

Some interesting properties are directly derived.

Proposition 2.2 *If Φ is a convex function, then*

1. *The directional derivative always exists, being finite or $+\infty$.*
2. $\partial\Phi(\zeta, \zeta) = 0$.
3. $\partial\Phi(\zeta, \zeta') \le \Phi(\zeta') - \Phi(\zeta)$,
4. *If Φ is nonnegative, a useful bound for the efficiency is*

$$eff_{\Phi}(\zeta) \ge 1 + \frac{\inf_{\zeta'} \partial\Phi(\zeta, \zeta')}{\Phi(\zeta)}.$$

Proof

1. If Φ is convex then the function

$$\frac{\Phi[(1-\epsilon)\zeta + \epsilon\zeta'] - \Phi(\zeta)}{\epsilon}$$

is increasing for $\epsilon \in (0, 1)$. In particular, let $0 < \epsilon_1 < \epsilon_2 < 1$, then

$$\begin{aligned}\frac{\Phi[(1-\epsilon_1)\zeta + \epsilon_1\zeta'] - \Phi(\zeta)}{\epsilon_1} &= \frac{\Phi\left\{\frac{\epsilon_1}{\epsilon_2}[(1-\epsilon_2)\zeta + \epsilon_2\zeta'] + (1-\frac{\epsilon_1}{\epsilon_2})\zeta\right\} - \Phi(\zeta)}{\epsilon_1} \\ &\le \frac{\frac{\epsilon_1}{\epsilon_2}\Phi[(1-\epsilon_2)\zeta + \epsilon_2\zeta'] + (1-\frac{\epsilon_1}{\epsilon_2})\Phi(\zeta) - \Phi(\zeta)}{\epsilon_1} \\ &= \frac{\{\Phi[(1-\epsilon_2)\zeta + \epsilon_2\zeta'] - \Phi(\zeta)\}}{\epsilon_2}.\end{aligned}$$

The limit of a continuous increasing function, which in this case is the directional derivative, exists and may be finite or infinity.
2. It is actually in the direction of $\zeta - \zeta = 0$.
3. Using the convexity of the criterion function,

$$\begin{aligned}\partial\Phi(\zeta, \zeta') &= \lim_{\epsilon\to 0^+} \frac{\Phi[(1-\epsilon)\zeta + \epsilon\zeta'] - \Phi(\zeta)}{\epsilon} \\ &\le \lim_{\epsilon\to 0^+} \frac{(1-\epsilon)\Phi(\zeta) + \epsilon\Phi(\zeta') - \Phi(\zeta)}{\epsilon} \\ &= \Phi(\zeta') - \Phi(\zeta).\end{aligned}$$

4. It is a direct consequence of previous result. The inequality keeps for the following infimum,

$$\inf_{\zeta'} \partial\Phi(\zeta, \zeta') \le \inf_{\zeta'} \{\Phi(\zeta') - \Phi(\zeta)\} = \Phi(\zeta^\star) - \Phi(\zeta),$$

where $\zeta^\star$ is the Φ-optimal design. Then, dividing by $\Phi(\zeta)$ (if positive),

$$\frac{\inf_{\zeta'} \partial\Phi(\zeta, \zeta')}{\Phi(\zeta)} \leq \frac{\Phi(\zeta^\star)}{\Phi(\zeta)} - 1 = \text{eff}_\Phi(\zeta) - 1.$$

□

Since $\mathcal{M}$ is within the cone of the nonnegative definite matrices in the Euclidean space of the symmetric matrices, the usual concept of *differentiability* applies here.

Proposition 2.3 *If Φ is differentiable on $\mathcal{M}$, then*

$$\partial\Phi(M, N) = tr[\nabla\Phi(M)(N - M)],$$

where $tr(A^T B)$ is the scalar product with matrix notation.

Proof Using the Taylor expansion,

$$\begin{aligned}\Phi[(1-\epsilon)M + \epsilon N] &= \Phi[M + \epsilon(N - M)] \\ &= \Phi(M) + \sum_{i,j} \left(\frac{\partial\Phi}{\partial m_{ij}}\right)_M \epsilon(n_{ij} - m_{ij}) + o(\epsilon).\end{aligned}$$

Then,

$$\begin{aligned}\partial\Phi(M, N) &= \lim_{\epsilon \to 0^+} \frac{\sum_{i,j} \left(\frac{\partial\Phi}{\partial m_{ij}}\right)_M \epsilon(n_{ij} - m_{ij}) + o(\epsilon)}{\epsilon} \\ &= \text{tr}[\nabla\Phi(M)(N - M)].\end{aligned}$$

□

Corollary 2.1 *The function Φ is differentiable on $\mathcal{M}$ if, and only if, $\partial\Phi(M, N)$ is linear on the second argument.*

This may be used as definition of a differentiable function. As a matter of fact, a function Φ defined in Ξ is called differentiable at ζ if the directional derivative is linear in any direction, ζ',

$$\partial\Phi(\zeta, \zeta') = \int_\chi \partial\Phi(\zeta, \zeta_x)\zeta'(dx).$$

As mentioned above, Kiefer and Wolfowitz (1960) provided a particular equivalence theorem, which was generalized in an elegant way by Whittle (1973). We show Whittle's version adapted for a better understanding.

Theorem 2.1 (General Equivalence Theorem, GET) *If Φ is convex on Ξ, the three conditions are equivalent:*

(i) $\Phi(\zeta^\star) = \min_{\zeta\in\Xi} \Phi(\zeta)$.
(ii) $\inf_{\zeta'\in\Xi} \partial\Phi(\zeta^\star, \zeta') = \max_{\zeta\in\Xi} \inf_{\zeta'\in\Xi} \partial\Phi(\zeta, \zeta')$.
(iii) $\inf_{\zeta'\in\Xi} \partial\Phi(\zeta^\star, \zeta') = 0$.

Moreover, if Φ is differentiable, then condition (ii) is satisfied if $\partial\Phi(\zeta^\star, \xi_x) = 0,\ x \in S_{\zeta^\star}$, where ξ_x corresponds to the Dirac measure at point x. This is a condition much easier to be checked.

Proof Since f is continuous and χ is compact, there exists a Φ-optimal design $\zeta^\star$ that satisfies (i). It is enough to prove this is the only one satisfying the three conditions.

By optimality $\partial\Phi(\zeta^\star, \zeta') \geq 0$ for any $\zeta' \in \Xi$. Thus, $\inf_{\zeta'\in\Xi} \partial\Phi(\zeta^\star, \zeta') \geq 0$, which is reached since $\partial\Phi(\zeta^\star, \zeta^\star) = 0$. Therefore, this design satisfies (iii).

On the other hand $\inf_{\zeta'\in\Xi} \partial\Phi(\zeta, \zeta') \leq \partial\Phi(\zeta, \zeta) = 0$ for any ζ, which is reached at least for $\zeta^\star$. Thus (ii) is also satisfied.

Finally, we need to prove that only optimal designs satisfy these conditions. Let ζ be nonoptimal. Then there exists ζ'' such that $\Phi(\zeta'') < \Phi(\zeta)$. Then $\partial\Phi(\zeta, \zeta'') \leq \Phi(\zeta'') - \Phi(\zeta) < 0$ and $\inf_{\zeta'\in\Xi} \partial\Phi(\zeta, \zeta') < 0$. And therefore, only an optimal design may satisfy (ii) and (iii). This ends the proof of the equivalence of the three conditions.

Additionally, if Φ is differentiable, then

$$\int_\chi \partial\Phi(\zeta^\star, \zeta_x)\zeta^\star(dx) = \partial\Phi(\zeta^\star, \zeta^\star) = 0.$$

But $\partial\Phi(\zeta^\star, \zeta_x) \geq 0$, thus the directional derivative should vanish at the support points. □

Remark 2.6

- The equivalence theorem can be applied just to approximate designs. Atkinson et al. (2007b) provided an example (9.4) where a D-optimal exact design does not satisfy the equivalence theorem.
- If the optimality is restricted to a convex subset of Ξ, say Ξ_R, the GET is still valid checking the directional derivative in all the directions of this set. It is easy to check that all the previous statements and proofs remain valid exchanging Ξ with Ξ_R. This result may be useful, for example, for marginally restricted designs (see, e.g., Sects. 6.4, 6.5, and 6.6) or, when the designs have to have some weight at some points, for example, for official regulatory requirements.
- From now on we assume finite support designs and use the symbol ξ (pdf) instead of ζ (measure) without loss of generality (see Appendix F.4).

2.6.1 Equivalence Theorem for Differentiable Criteria

The following lemma summarizes three properties for a differentiable criterion.

Lemma 2.1 *Let Φ be differentiable on $\mathcal{M}$, then*

(i) $\partial\Phi[M(\xi), M(\xi')] = \sum_x \partial\Phi[M(\xi), M(\xi_x)]\xi'(x)$.
(ii) $\partial\Phi[M(\xi), M(\xi'))] = \operatorname{tr}\left\{\nabla\Phi[M(\xi)][M(\xi') - M(\xi)]\right\}$ *(from Proposition 2.3).*
(iii) $\partial\Phi[M(\xi^\star), f(x)f^T(x)] \geq 0$, *for any* $x \in \chi$.

In this case the GET has a friendly version based on the so-called *sensitivity function*, that is, the directional derivative in the direction of one-point designs,

$$\begin{aligned}\psi(x,\xi) &= \partial\Phi[M(\xi), f(x)f^T(x)]\\ &= f^T(x)\nabla\Phi[M(\xi)]f(x) - \operatorname{tr}M(\xi)\nabla\Phi[M(\xi)].\end{aligned}$$

Then the GET establishes that ξ^* is Φ-optimal if and only if $\psi(x, \xi^*) \geq 0,\ x \in \chi$. The equality is reached for $x \in S_{\xi^\star}$.

Taking into account there is a bound for the number of support points, the so-called *checking condition* can be used to compute analytic optimal designs. If $\xi^\star$ is Φ-optimal, then

$$\psi(z, \xi^\star) = 0,\ z \in S_\xi^\star$$

$$\left(\frac{\partial\psi(x,\xi^\star)}{\partial x}\right)_{x=z} = 0,\ z \in S_\xi^\star \cap \operatorname{Int}(\chi),$$

where $\operatorname{Int}(\chi)$ stands for the topological interior set of the design space χ. These are necessary conditions that may help to compute a candidate for being the optimal design. Then the GET should be checked to see whether it is optimal or no. Let us show how this works in a simple case.

Example 2.8 For a two-parameter model we may guess that the optimal design is going to be a two-point design. Actually, this happens usually in practice. Thus, a general candidate will be

$$\xi = \left\{\begin{matrix} x_1 & x_2 \\ 1-p & p\end{matrix}\right\},$$

and then the three variables $x_1, x_2 \in \chi$ and $0 \leq p \leq 1$ have to be optimized. From the checking condition there are two equations

$$\psi(x_1, \xi) = 0,\ \psi(x_2, \xi) = 0$$

and 0, 1, or 2 additional equations

$$\left(\frac{\partial \psi(x,\xi)}{\partial x}\right)_{x=x_1} = 0, \quad \left(\frac{\partial \psi(x,\xi)}{\partial x}\right)_{x=x_2} = 0.$$

Of course, the objective function Φ restricted to two-point designs can be minimized directly, but these equations may help.

Example 2.9 In what follows the checking condition will be used for a quadratic model,

$$E[y] = \theta^T f(x) = \theta_1 + \theta_2 x + \theta_3 x^2, \sigma^2(x) = 1, \; x \in \chi = [-1, 2].$$

here, $f(x) = (1, x, x^2)^T$, and the FIM is

$$\begin{aligned} M(\xi) &= \sum_{x\in[-1,2]} f(x) f^T(x)\xi(x) \\ &= \sum_{x\in[-1,2]} \xi(x) \begin{pmatrix} 1 & x & x^2 \\ x & x^2 & x^3 \\ x^2 & x^3 & x^4 \end{pmatrix} \end{aligned}$$

Assume the D-optimal design is of the type:

$$\xi = \begin{Bmatrix} -1 & z & 2 \\ 1/3 & 1/3 & 1/3 \end{Bmatrix}.$$

This seems to be a strong assumption since we only know the D-optimal design has at most $\frac{3\times 4}{2} = 6$ points (D-optimality is strictly convex), but we may take into account that frequently the D-optimal design has as many support points as parameters and the extremes of the interval are between them. Then, the fact that if the D-optimal design has m points in its support then they have to be equally weighted is used. This means the assumption is not so strong. In any case, if the design found optimizing value z is not optimal, we should start to relax the conditions, for example, not assuming both extreme points are in the support.

The value $z^\star = 0.5$ maximizes the determinant,

$$\det M(\xi) = \frac{1}{3}\left(-z^2 + z + 2\right)^2,$$

giving the design

$$\xi^\star = \begin{Bmatrix} -1 & 0.5 & 2 \\ 1/3 & 1/3 & 1/3 \end{Bmatrix}.$$

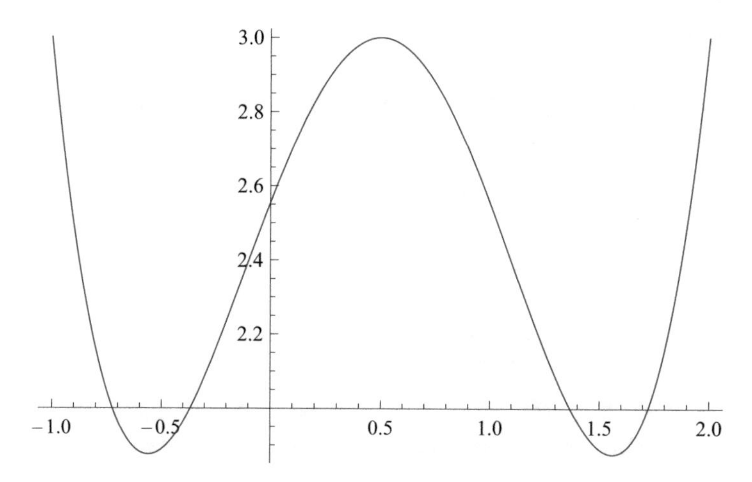

Fig. 2.9 Function $d(x, \xi^\star)$

The design $\xi^\star$ will be D-optimal if the following function is under 3,

$$
\begin{aligned}
d(x, \xi^\star) &= f^T(x) M^{-1}(\xi^\star) f(x) \\
&= 0.89 \left(x^2 - 3.43x + 3.3\right)\left(x^2 + 1.43x + 0.87\right).
\end{aligned}
$$

This can be proved analytically and moreover Fig. 2.9 shows it.

2.6.2 *Efficiency Bounds*

As seen previously, this is a very general bound for any convex criterion,

$$
\text{eff}_\Phi(\xi) \geq 1 + \frac{\inf_{\xi'} \partial\Phi(\xi, \xi')}{\Phi(\xi)}.
$$

If the criterion is differentiable, this bound is much more tractable,

$$
\text{eff}_\Phi(\xi) \geq 1 + \frac{\inf_x \partial\Phi(\xi, \xi_x)}{\Phi(\xi)}, \tag{2.5}
$$

where $\psi(x, \xi) = \partial\Phi(\xi, \xi_x)$ is sometimes so-called sensitivity function.

This bound is now individualized for some of the criteria mentioned above. In particular, the bounds are considered for nonsingular designs (information matrices).

D-optimality

The following definition, which is inverse positive homogeneous, will be used for the bounds,

$$\Phi_D(\xi) = \det M^{-1/m}(\xi),$$

The bound (2.5) for this criterion is then

$$\text{eff}_D(\xi) \geq 2 - \frac{\max_x d(x, \xi)}{m},$$

where $d(x, \xi) = f^T(x)M^{-1}(\xi)f(x)$ is sometimes called generalized variance.

For D-optimality there is a sharper bound for any design, due to Atwood (1969),

$$\text{eff}_D(\xi) \geq \frac{m}{\max_x d(x, \xi)}.$$

Proof Using Proposition II.12 from Pázman (1986), let L be a matrix such that $LM(\xi)L^T = I$ and a diagonal matrix, Λ, with $LM(\xi_D^\star)L^T = \Lambda$. Define $g(x) = Lf(x)$, $x \in \chi$. Then $N(\xi) = \sum_x \xi(x)g(x)g^T(x) = LM(\xi)L^T = I$ is the FIM for the linear model defined by $g(x)$. Thus, $1 = \det N(\xi) = \det M(\xi) \det^2 L$.

Therefore, we can assume $M(\xi) = I$ without loss of generality. Then $d(x, \xi) = f^T(x)f(x)$ and for the D-optimal design $\xi_D^\star$,

$$\max_x d(x, \xi) \geq \int_\xi d(x, \xi)\xi_D^\star(dx) = \int_\xi f^T(x)f(x)\xi_D^\star(x)dx = \text{tr}M(\xi_D^\star).$$

The arithmetic-geometric mean inequality establishes that

$$\left(\frac{\det M(\xi)}{\det M(\xi_D^\star)}\right)^{1/m} = \det M^{-1/m}(\xi_D^\star) \geq \frac{m}{\text{tr}M(\xi_D^\star)} \geq \frac{m}{\max_x d(x, \xi)}.$$

□

$\mathbf{D}_s$-optimality

Let ξ be a nonsingular design and denote

$$d_s(x, \xi) = f^T(x)M^{-1}(\xi)f(x) - f_2^T(x)[M(\xi)]_{22}^{-1} f_2(x),$$

where $f^T(x) = (f_1^T(x), f_2^T(x))$ for $f_1^T(x)$ corresponding to the s first parameters. After some algebra the gradient is

$$\nabla \Phi_{D_s}[M(\xi)] = \frac{1}{s}\Phi_{D_s}[M(\xi)]\left[\begin{pmatrix} 0 & 0 \\ 0 & [M(\xi)]_{22}^{-1} \end{pmatrix} - M^{-1}(\xi)\right].$$

Therefore, the directional derivative in the direction of a one-point design is

$$\begin{aligned} \partial\Phi_{D_s}[M(\xi), f(x)f^T(x)] &= \text{tr}\nabla\Phi_{D_s}[M(\xi)][f(x)f^T(x) - M(\xi)] \\ &= \frac{1}{s}\Phi_{D_s}[M(\xi)][s - d_s(x, \xi)] \end{aligned}$$

and therefore

$$\text{eff}_{D_s}(\xi) \geq 2 - \frac{\max_x d_s(x, \xi)}{s}.$$

L-optimality

The following definition, which is inverse positive homogeneous, will be used for the bound (2.5),

$$\Phi_L(\xi) = \text{tr}WM^{-1}(\xi),$$

where W is positive definite. Then,

$$\text{eff}_L(\xi) \geq 2 - \frac{\max_x f^T(x)M^{-1}WM^{-1}(\xi)f(x)}{\text{tr}WM^{-1}(\xi)}.$$

This is valid for A-optimality for $W = I$ and also for I-optimality with $W = \int_S f(x)f^T(x)\mu(dx)$ and

$$\Phi_I(\xi) = \int_S f^T(x)M^{-1}(\xi)f(x)\mu(dx) = \text{tr}\left[\int_S f(x)f^T(x)\mu(dx)\right]M^{-1}(\xi),$$

where S is a set of experimental conditions with interest in making predictions and μ is a probability measure on S describing the distributed interest in predicting at values of S.

E-optimality

This is a minimax criterion and therefore it is not differentiable. This introduces some complexity to find an operative bound for the efficiency, but it is still possible.

The definition, which is inverse positive homogeneous, is

$$\Phi_E(\xi) = \lambda_{min}^{-1}[M(\xi)].$$

Then

$$\text{eff}_E(\xi) \geq 2 - \frac{\max_x \sum_{i=1}^{a} \pi_i P_i^T f(x) f^T(x) P_i}{\lambda_{min}[M(\xi)]},$$

where $\lambda_{min}[M(\xi)]P_i = M(\xi)P_i$, a is the algebraic multiplicity of $\lambda_{min}[M(\xi)]$ and there exists a probability measure satisfying that $\sum_{i=1}^{a} \pi_i = 1$, $0 \leq \pi_i \leq 1$. The problem is finding this probability measure for each design. Of course, if $\lambda_{min}[M(\xi)]$ has multiplicity 1, there is no problem.

Example 2.10 Revisiting Examples 2.4 and 2.5, bounds for the efficiency of the designs considered are provided for each of the four criteria given in the examples. Then optimal designs are computed for the simple linear regression model and the exact efficiencies are compared with the bounds. Table 2.2 shows the bounds for the efficiencies of the four designs. The negative numbers are actually the bounds computed with the formula provided. Since the efficiency is always positive by definition, those bounds are useless, meaning they are far from the optimum. As a matter of fact, these efficiencies are sharp, just near the optimal designs. In any case the Atwood bound is much better than the general one.

Let us compute now the optimal designs for the different criteria using some of the tools introduced so far.

D-optimal Design

If we guess the D-optimal design is a two-point design with the two extreme points 0 and 1, then we know the weights have to be equal,

$$\xi_D = \left\{ \begin{matrix} 0 & 1 \\ 0.5 & 0.5 \end{matrix} \right\}$$

Table 2.2 Bounds of the efficiencies versus actual efficiencies (between brackets)

Design	ξ	$\xi_{12}^{\star}$	$\xi_{12}^{\star\star}$	$\xi_{12}^{\star\star\star}$
D-efficiency bound	0.21 (0.74)	−0.01(0.72)	0.43 (0.79)	0.48 (0.75)
D-efficiency Atwood bound	0.55 (0.74)	0.49 (0.72)	0.63 (0.79)	0.65 (0.75)
A-efficiency bound	−0.91(0.54)	−1.35(0.49)	−0.47(0.62)	−0.35(0.58)
c-efficiency bound	−0.58(0.55)	−1.01(0.52)	−0.14(0.63)	−0.04(0.57)
E-efficiency bound	−1.08(0.49)	−1.53(0.45)	−0.63(0.57)	−0.49(0.54)

Let us check with the equivalence theorem whether this design is D-optimal. All we have to do is to prove that

$$\max_{x\in[0,1]} d(x, \xi_D) = 2.$$

But

$$d(x, \xi_D) = f^T(x)M^{-1}(\xi)f(x) = (1, x)\begin{pmatrix} 1 & 0.5 \\ 0.5 & 0.5 \end{pmatrix}\begin{pmatrix} 1 \\ x \end{pmatrix}$$
$$= 2 - 4x + 4x^2.$$

And the maximum, 2, is reached at $x = 0$ and 1. Thus, this is actually the D-optimal design.

A-optimal Design

In a similar way, assuming the A-optimal design is of the type,

$$\xi_A = \begin{Bmatrix} 0 & 1 \\ 1 - p & p \end{Bmatrix},$$

the trace of the inverse of the FIM is reached at $p^\star = \sqrt{2} - 1$. The GET says this is optimal if

$$\max_{x\in[0,1]} f^T(x)M^{-2}(\xi_A)f(x) = \mathrm{tr}M^{-2}(\xi_A).$$

But, $f^T(x)M^{-2}(\xi_A)f(x) = \left(10 + 7\sqrt{2}\right)(x - 1)x + 2\sqrt{2} + 3$ and its maximum, $\mathrm{tr}M^{-2}(\xi_A) = 3 + 2\sqrt{2}$, is reached at 0 and 1. Thus,

$$\xi_A = \begin{Bmatrix} 0 & 1 \\ 2 - \sqrt{2} & \sqrt{2} - 1 \end{Bmatrix}.$$

E-optimal Design

Assuming again a two-point design at the extreme points, the biggest eigenvalue of the inverse of the FIM is

$$\frac{\sqrt{5p^2 - 2p + 1} + p + 1}{2p - 2p^2},$$

which is minimized at $p^\star = 2/5$. The inverse of the FIM is then

$$\begin{pmatrix} 1 & 2/5 \\ 2/5 & 2/5 \end{pmatrix}.$$

The minimum eigenvalue is $1/5$ and the corresponding eigenvector is $(-1/2, 1)^T$. Thus, the GET stablishes this design is E-optimal if and only if (Sect. 2.6.2)

$$\max_x \sum_{i=1}^{a} \pi_i P_i^T f(x) f^T(x) P_i = \lambda_{min}[M(\xi_E)],$$

where the multiplicity of $\lambda_{min}[M(\xi_E)] = 1/5$ is 1 and $P_i = (-1/2, 1)^T$. Actually,

$$P_i^T f(x) f^T(x) P_i = (-1/2, 1) \begin{pmatrix} 1 & x \\ x & x^2 \end{pmatrix} \begin{pmatrix} -1/2 \\ 1 \end{pmatrix} = 4/5(1/2 - x)^2,$$

which reaches the maximum at $\lambda_{min}[M(\xi_E)] = 1/5$.

c-Optimal Design

The c-optimal design can be easily computed using the Elfving graph procedure. Figure 2.10 shows how vector $c^T = (0, 1)$ determines the c-optimal design,

$$\xi_c = \begin{Bmatrix} 0 & 1 \\ 0.5 & 0.5 \end{Bmatrix},$$

and there is no need to check optimality at all.

Table 2.2 shows the actual efficiencies of the four designs for different criterion functions. They are much larger than those of Table 2.2.

2.7 Algorithms

In the area of OED much effort has been devoted to outlining different statistical problems, giving theoretical results as much general as possible. Analytic results are possible mainly for just one variable and a few parameters in the model. In practice, several variables and parameters are involved in the model and providing analytic solutions is not affordable any more. Then efficient algorithms are welcome for computing designs in practice.

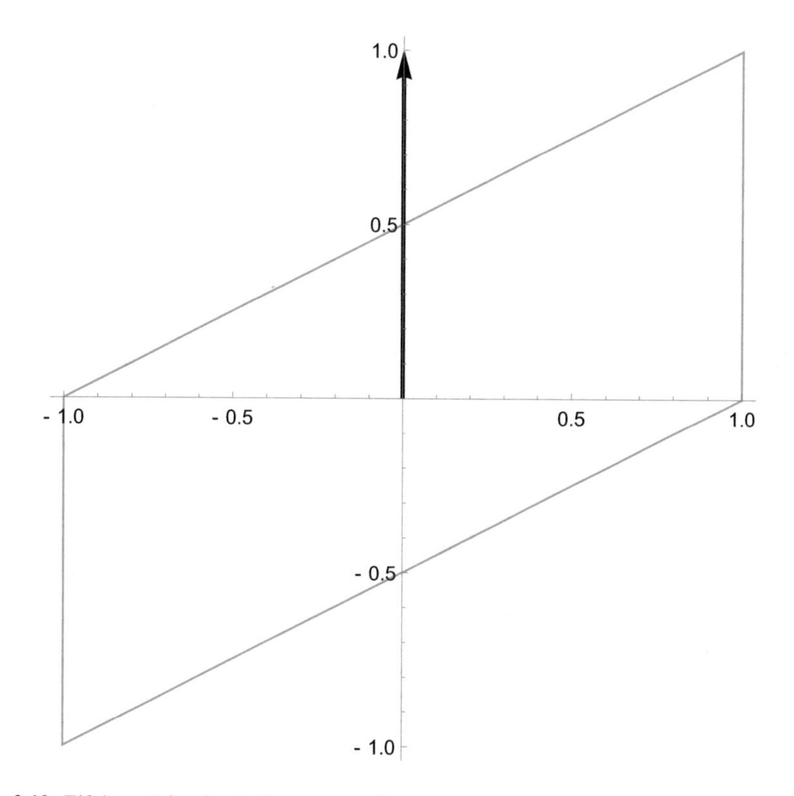

Fig. 2.10 Elfving set for simple linear regression

2.7.1 Fedorov–Wynn Algorithm

The so-called Fedorov–Wynn algorithm (Fedorov, 1972; Wynn, 1970) has an interesting origin. Fedorov's book was first published in Russian and independently about the same time Wynn published a paper in 1970. Both works offered a *first-order algorithm* for computing optimal designs using the equivalence theorem. Later on, when the Fedorov's book was translated into English, it came out to the international community that basically the same procedure was there. This algorithm has been very much used and adapted in the literature of optimal experimental design construction. I know both authors well and I can credit they are good friends and none of them claims for been the first as it happens frequently in science. I believe this is a good example for scientists.

The criterion function Φ is assumed differentiable, but the algorithm can be formulated for some non-differentiable criteria as well. The algorithm starts with an initial nonsingular design and after s steps the design ξ_s is improved adding a new point or giving more weight to an existing point,

$$\xi_{s+1} = (1 - \alpha_s)\xi_s + \alpha_s \xi_{x_s},$$

where

$$x_s = \arg\min_{x\in\chi} f^T(x)\nabla\Phi[M(\xi_s)]f(x).$$

The steps may be $\alpha_s = 1/(s+1)$, or they can be optimized using the criterion function,

$$\alpha_s = \arg\min_{\alpha\in[0,1]} \Phi\left\{M[(1-\alpha)\xi_s + \alpha\xi_{x_s}]\right\}.$$

The stopping rule comes from the GET efficiency bound (2.5) for differentiable criteria,

$$\text{eff}_\Phi[M(\xi_s)] \geq 1 + \frac{\min_x \psi(x,\xi_s)}{\Phi[M(\xi_s)]}.$$

The following theorems proves the convergence of the algorithm under certain conditions of the criterion function. This previous and instrumental lemma has to be proved first.

Lemma 2.2 *Let Φ be a criterion function, ξ_1 and ξ_2 two designs, and $\xi_\alpha = (1-\alpha)\xi_2 + \alpha\xi_2$ with $\alpha \in [0,1]$, then*

$$\left.\frac{\partial}{\partial\alpha}\Phi[M(\xi_\alpha)]\right|_{\alpha=0} = \partial\Phi[M(\xi_1), M(\xi_2)].$$

Proof

$$\begin{aligned}
&\left.\frac{\partial}{\partial\alpha}\Phi[M(\xi_\alpha)]\right|_{\alpha=0} \\
&= \lim_{\alpha\to 0}\lim_{\varepsilon\to 0} \frac{\Phi[(1-\alpha-\varepsilon)M(\xi_1) + (\alpha+\varepsilon)M(\xi_2)] - \Phi[(1-\alpha)M(\xi_1 + \alpha M(\xi_2)]}{\varepsilon} \\
&= \lim_{\varepsilon\to 0} \frac{\Phi[(1-\varepsilon)M(\xi_1) + (\varepsilon)M(\xi_2)] - \Phi[M(\xi_1)]}{\varepsilon} \\
&= \partial\Phi[M(\xi 1), M(\xi_2)].
\end{aligned}$$

□

Theorem 2.2 *If Φ is a criterion function such that*

1. *Φ is bounded below and achieves its minimum at $M(\xi^\star)$.*
2. *Φ has bounded second-order derivatives, that is, there exists $0 < B < \infty$, such that $|\partial^2\Phi/\partial m_{ij}\partial m_{rt}| \leq B$.*
3. *Let $\{\alpha_s\}_{s=0}^\infty$ be a sequence such that $\lim_{s\to\infty}\alpha_s = 0$, $\sum_{s=0}^\infty \alpha_s = \infty$ and $\sum_{s=0}^\infty \alpha_s^2 < \infty$,*

then $\lim_{s\to\infty}\Phi[M(\xi_s)] = \Phi[M(\xi^\star)]$.

Proof The information matrix of the design at step $s+1$ of the algorithm is

$$M(\xi_{s+1}) = M(\xi_s) + \alpha_s[f(x_s)f^T(x_s) - \sum_{x\in\chi} f(x)f^T(x)\xi_s(x)].$$

If ξ_s is not Φ-optimal, then the following inequality holds:

$$\begin{aligned}\partial\Phi[M(\xi_s), f(x_s)f^T(x_s)] &= \inf_x \partial\Phi[M(\xi_s), f(x)f^T(x)] \\ &= \inf_{\xi'} \partial\Phi[M(\xi_s), M(\xi')] \\ &< \max_{\xi} \inf_{\xi'} \partial\Phi[M(\xi), M(\xi')] \\ &= \inf_{\xi'} \partial\Phi[M(\xi^\star), M(\xi')] = 0,\end{aligned}$$

where the second equality comes from the differentiability and the last two from the equivalence theorem taking into account the choice of x_s in the algorithm.

The Taylor expansion in α_s provides

$$\begin{aligned}\Phi[M(\xi_{s+1})] &= \Phi[M(\xi_s)] + \alpha_s \left.\frac{\partial}{\partial\alpha_s}\Phi[M(\xi_{s+1})]\right|_{\alpha_s=0} + o(\alpha_s) \\ &= \Phi[M(\xi_s)] + \alpha_s\partial\Phi[M(\xi_s), f(x_s)f^T(x_s)] + o(\alpha_s),\end{aligned}$$

where the partial derivative has been computed taking into account the linearity of the directional derivative (Wu & Wynn, 1978) given in Lemma 2.2,

$$\left.\frac{\partial}{\partial\alpha_s}\Phi[M(\xi_{s+1})]\right|_{\alpha_s=0} = \partial\Phi[M(\xi_s), f(x_s)f^T(x_s)].$$

Thus, for small values of α_s then $\Phi[M(\xi_{s+1})] - \Phi[M(\xi_s)] \leq 0$, with equality only if ξ_s is optimal. Let $W_s = \partial\Phi[M(\xi_s), f(x_s)f^T(x_s)]$. Since $\partial\Phi[M(\xi_s), f(x_s)f^T(x_s)] < 0$, the series $R_s = \sum_{i=0}^s \alpha_i W_i$ decreases monotonically. Using the Taylor expansion recursively

$$\Phi[M(\xi_{s+1})] = \Phi[M(\xi_1)] + R_s + \sum_{i=0}^{s} \alpha_i^2 k_i \geq \Phi[M(\xi^\star)],$$

where the second derivative k_i is bounded, $|k_i| \leq B$, $i = 1, 2, \ldots$ Convergence follows from this, the monotonicity of R_s and the convergence of $\sum_{s=0}^\infty \alpha_s^2$.

Finally, it has to be proved that the convergence is actually to the optimal design. Assume that $\lim_{s\to\infty} \Phi[M(\xi_s)] = \Phi[M(\tilde{\xi})] > \Phi[M(\xi^\star)] + d$ for some $d > 0$. From the asymptotic monotonicity of $\Phi[M(\xi_s)]$, there exists s_0 and $\varepsilon > 0$ such that $W_s < -\varepsilon$ for $s > s_0$ and then $R_s = \sum_{i=0}^{s_0} \alpha_i W_i + \sum_{i=s_0+1}^{s} \alpha_i W_i < \sum_{i=0}^{s_0} \alpha_i W_i -$

$\varepsilon \sum_{i=s_0+1}^{s} \alpha_i$. Thus, $R_s \longrightarrow -\infty$ and $\Phi[M(\xi_s)] \longrightarrow -\infty$ as $s \to \infty$; this is in contradiction with the assumption of Φ being bounded below.

□

Unfortunately, the hypothesis of Theorem 2.2 does not apply to D- or L-optimality: indeed, the second-order derivative is unbounded. This causes much trouble for proving convergence of general step-length algorithms, see especially Wu and Wynn (1978). A proof of convergence for D-optimality can be found in (Fedorov and Hackl, 1997, p. 48, Theorem 3.1.1).

2.7.2 *Multiplicative Algorithm for D- and G-optimality for a Finite Design Space*

Assuming a finite design space is not restrictive at all if we take into account that in practice a few decimal figures are considered for the support points. Of course, if the discretization produces a very big set of possible design points, then the procedures based on finite search sets may not be efficient. Let $\chi = \{x_1, \ldots, x_N\}$ be a discretized design space.

- Let ξ_0 be an initial design such that $\xi_0(x_i) > 0,\ i = 1, 2, \ldots, N$.
- Given ξ_s, constructed at step s, we define

$$\xi_{s+1}(x_i) = \xi_s(x_i)\frac{d(x_i, \xi_s)}{m}, i = 1, 2, \ldots, n.$$

- A stopping rule based on the efficiency bound can be used, $\text{eff}_D(\xi) \geq \frac{m}{\max_x d(x,\xi)} \geq \delta$ (e.g., 0.99).

Remark 2.7

1. A proof of the convergence of this algorithm can be found in Pázman (1986), p. 139, Proposition V.6, and, in a more general setting, in Yu (2010).
2. The design obtained in step 2. is a design since for any design ξ and any design space

$$\begin{aligned}\sum_{x\in\chi} \xi(x)d(x, \xi) &= \sum_{x\in\chi} \xi(x) f^T(x)M^{-1}(\xi) f(x)\\ &= \text{tr}\left[M^{-1}(\xi)\sum_{x\in\chi} \xi(x) f(x) f^T(x)\right]\\ &= \text{tr}[M^{-1}(\xi)M(\xi)] = \text{tr}I_m = m.\end{aligned}$$

Example 2.11 Let consider simple linear regression with a finite design space. If there is interest in just one decimal figure, then the design space can be assumed as $\chi = \{0, 0.1, 0.2, \ldots, 0.9, 1\}$. Let ξ_0 be the equal weights design at these points. Its information matrix is

$$M(\xi_0) = \sum_{i=0}^{10} \frac{1}{11} \begin{pmatrix} 1 & i/10 \\ i/10 & i^2/10^2 \end{pmatrix} = \begin{pmatrix} 1 & 1/2 \\ 1/2 & 7/20 \end{pmatrix},$$

with inverse

$$M^{-1}(\xi_0) = \begin{pmatrix} 7/2 & -5 \\ -5 & 10 \end{pmatrix},$$

and for $x_i = i/10,\ i = 0, \ldots, 10,$

$$\begin{aligned} d(x_i, \xi_0) &= (1, x_i) M^{-1}(\xi_0) \begin{pmatrix} 1 \\ x_i \end{pmatrix} \\ &= \frac{7}{2} - 10x_i + 10x_i^2 \\ &= \frac{7}{2} - i + \frac{i^2}{10}, i = 0, 1, \ldots, 10. \end{aligned}$$

At first step,

$$\begin{aligned} \xi_1(x_i) &= \xi_0(x_i) \frac{d(x_i, \xi_0)}{2},\ x_i = i/10, i = 0, 1, \ldots, 10 = \frac{1}{11} \frac{\frac{7}{2} - i + \frac{i^2}{10}}{2} \\ &= \frac{35 - 10i + i^2}{220}, \end{aligned}$$

that is,

$$\xi_1 = \begin{Bmatrix} 0 & \frac{1}{10} & \frac{1}{5} & \frac{3}{10} & \frac{2}{5} & \frac{1}{2} & \frac{3}{5} & \frac{7}{10} & \frac{4}{5} & \frac{9}{10} & 1 \\ \frac{7}{22} & \frac{13}{55} & \frac{19}{110} & \frac{7}{55} & \frac{1}{10} & \frac{1}{11} & \frac{1}{10} & \frac{7}{55} & \frac{19}{110} & \frac{13}{55} & \frac{7}{22} \end{Bmatrix},$$

with $\text{eff}_D[M(\xi_1)] \geq 2 - \frac{\max_x d(x,\xi_1)}{2} = 0.25$. Figure 2.11 shows how far this design is from being D-optimal (all the points should be under 2).

After 14 iterations an efficiency greater than 99% is reached for the design:

$$\xi_{14} = \begin{Bmatrix} 0. & 0.1 & 0.2 & 0.3 & 0.4 \\ 0.48 & 0.021 & 0.0011 & 7.4 \times 10^{-5} & 1.1 \times 10^{-5} \end{matrix}$$

$$\begin{matrix} 0.5 & 0.6 & 0.7 & 0.8 & 0.9 & 1 \\ 5.5 \times 10^{-6} & 1.1 \times 10^{-5} & 7.4 \times 10^{-5} & 0.0011 & 0.021 & 0.48 \end{Bmatrix}$$

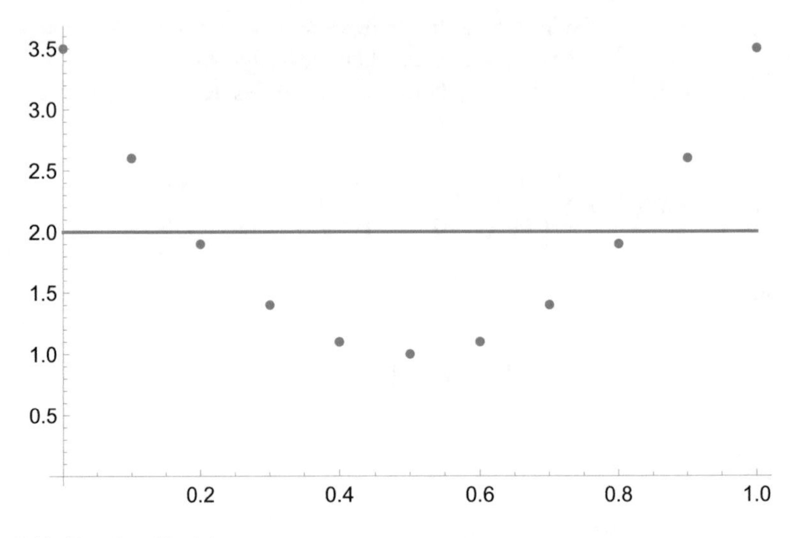

Fig. 2.11 Function $d(x, \xi_1)$

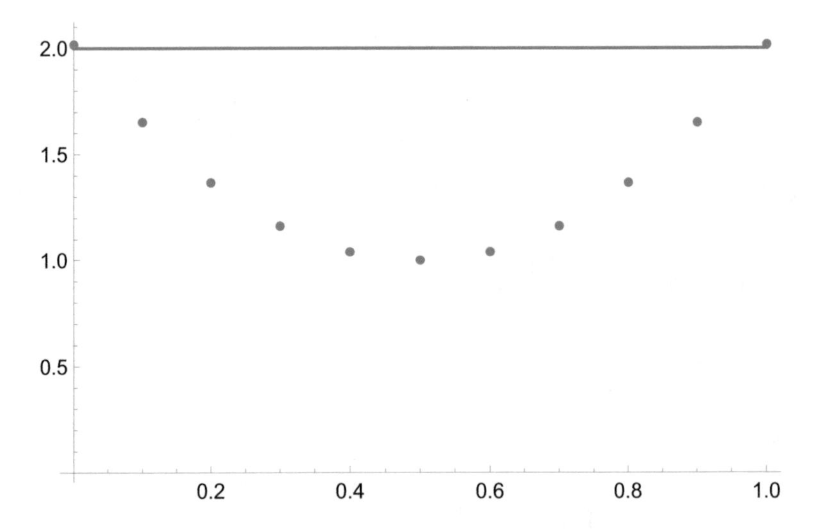

Fig. 2.12 Function $d(x, \xi_{14})$

The sensitivity function (Fig. 2.12) shows this design is almost optimal (points under 2). In these situations some of the points with a very small weight may be removed increasing the efficiency of the procedure. Actually, the D-optimal design is a two-point design with support points at the extremes (0 and 1) and equal weights, and that the sensitivity is equal to 2 at these points, which is approximately reflected in Fig. 2.12.

2.7.3 *Recursive Computation of the Determinant and the Inverse of a Matrix*

Previous algorithms and many others need to compute the inverse of the new information matrix at each step. This means an important computation burden and recursive formulae may speed up computation very much. Let the design built at step $s+1$ be

$$\xi_{s+1} = (1-\alpha)\xi_s + \alpha\xi_x,\ \alpha \in (0,1),$$

such that $\det M(\xi_s) \neq 0$. Then $\det M(\xi_{s+1}) \neq 0$ and:

$$M^{-1}(\xi_{s+1}) = \frac{1}{1-\alpha}\left\{M^{-1}(\xi_s) - \frac{\alpha M^{-1}(\xi_s) f(x) f^T(x) M^{-1}(\xi_s)}{1-\alpha+\alpha f^T(x) M^{-1}(\xi_s) f(x)}\right\}, \quad (2.6)$$

$$\det M^{-1}(\xi_{s+1}) = \frac{\det M^{-1}(\xi_s)}{(1-\alpha)^m}\left[1 - \frac{\alpha f^T(x) M^{-1}(\xi_s) f(x)}{1-\alpha+\alpha f^T(x) M^{-1}(\xi_s) f(x)}\right]. \quad (2.7)$$

$$d(x,\xi_{s+1}) = \frac{1}{1-\alpha}\left[d(x,\xi_s) - \frac{\alpha[f^T(x) M^{-1}(\xi_s) f(x_s)]^2}{1-\alpha+\alpha d(x,\xi_s)}\right]. \quad (2.8)$$

Formulae 2.6 and 2.7 are due to the Sherman–Morrison–Woodbury formulae.

Example 2.12 Simple linear regression,

$$E[y] = \theta^T f(x) = \theta_1 + \theta_2 x, \sigma^2(x) = 1,\ x \in \chi = [0,1],\ f(x) = (1,x)^T.$$

The information matrix is

$$\begin{aligned} M(\xi) &= \sum_{x\in[0,1]} f(x) f^T(x)\xi(x) \\ &= \sum_{x\in[0,1]} \xi(x)\begin{pmatrix} 1 & x \\ x & x^2 \end{pmatrix} \end{aligned}$$

The first-order algorithm is developed here step by step. Let an initial design be

$$\xi_0 = \begin{Bmatrix} 0 & 1 \\ 1/4 & 3/4 \end{Bmatrix}.$$

Its information matrix is

$$M(\xi_0) = \begin{pmatrix} 1 & 3/4 \\ 3/4 & 3/4 \end{pmatrix}, \det M(\xi_0) = 3/16,$$

and the inverse

$$M^{-1}(\xi_0) = \begin{pmatrix} 4 & -4 \\ -4 & 16/3 \end{pmatrix}.$$

The sensitivity function is computed,

$$\begin{aligned} d(x, \xi_0) &= f^T(x) M^{-1}(\xi_0) f(x) \\ &= (1, x) \begin{pmatrix} 4 & -4 \\ -4 & 16/3 \end{pmatrix} \begin{pmatrix} 1 \\ x \end{pmatrix} \\ &= 4 - 8x + \frac{16}{3} x^2, \end{aligned}$$

and a new design constructed

$$\xi_1 = \left(1 - \frac{1}{2}\right) \xi_0 + \frac{1}{2} \xi_{x_0} = \frac{1}{2} \xi_0 + \frac{1}{2} \xi_{x_0},$$

where

$$x_0 = \arg \max_{x \in [0,1]} 4 - 8x + \frac{16}{3} x^2 = 0.$$

Thus,

$$\xi_1 = \begin{Bmatrix} 0 & 1 \\ 5/8 & 3/8 \end{Bmatrix}.$$

The inverse of the information matrix is computed using the recursive equation (2.6),

$$\begin{aligned} M^{-1}(\xi_1) &= \frac{1}{1/2} \begin{pmatrix} 4 & -4 \\ -4 & 16/3 \end{pmatrix} \\ &\quad - \frac{1/2 \begin{pmatrix} 4 & -4 \\ -4 & 16/3 \end{pmatrix} \begin{pmatrix} 1 \\ 0 \end{pmatrix} (1, 0) \begin{pmatrix} 4 & -4 \\ -4 & 16/3 \end{pmatrix}}{1/2 + 4/2} \\ &= \begin{pmatrix} 8/5 & -8/5 \\ -8/15 & 64/15 \end{pmatrix}. \end{aligned}$$

and

$$d(x, \xi_1) = (1, x) \begin{pmatrix} 8/5 & -8/5 \\ -8/15 & 64/15 \end{pmatrix} \begin{pmatrix} 1 \\ x \end{pmatrix} = \frac{8}{5} - \frac{16}{5}x + \frac{64}{15}x^2$$

reaches the maximum at $x_1 = 1$. Therefore,

$$\xi_2 = 2/3\xi_1 + 1/3\xi_{x_1} = \begin{Bmatrix} 0 & 1 \\ 5/12 & 7/12 \end{Bmatrix}$$

with

$$M^{-1}(\xi_2) = \begin{pmatrix} 12/5 & -12/5 \\ -12/5 & 272/55 \end{pmatrix}.$$

Then

$$x_2 = \arg\max_x d(x, \xi_2) = \frac{12}{5} - \frac{24}{5}x + \frac{272}{55}x^2 = 1,$$

$$\xi_3 = 3/4\xi_2 + 1/4\xi_{x_2} = \begin{Bmatrix} 0 & 1 \\ 5/16 & 11/16 \end{Bmatrix}.$$

The algorithm goes on until the required efficiency bound is reached.

Nevertheless, in this particular case, after a while it seems that the optimal design may be,

$$\xi^\star = \begin{Bmatrix} 0 & 1 \\ 1/2 & 1/2 \end{Bmatrix}.$$

We always can check whether this design is actually D-optimal or not using the GET,

$$M(\xi^\star) = \begin{pmatrix} 1 & 1/2 \\ 1/2 & 1/2 \end{pmatrix}, \det M(\xi^\star) = 1/4, M^{-1}(\xi^\star) = \begin{pmatrix} 2 & -2 \\ -2 & 4 \end{pmatrix},$$

$$d(x, \xi^\star) = 2 - 4x + 4x^2,$$

whose maximum is 2, reached at $x = 0$ and $x = 1$. Thus, it is a D-optimal design. Function $d(x, \xi^\star)$ in Fig. 2.13 remains under 2 (number of support points, which is reached at the two design points). Remember the sensitivity function for D-optimality, $m - d(x, \xi^\star) \geq 0, \; x \in \chi$.

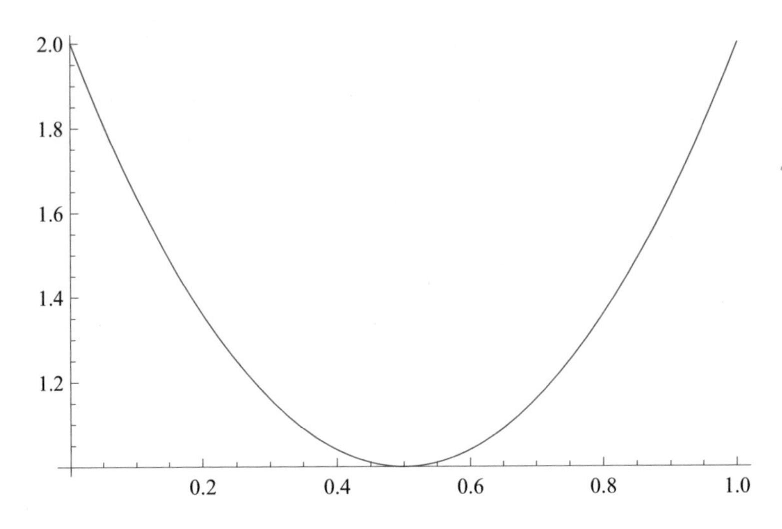

Fig. 2.13 Function $d(x, \xi^{\star})$ for simple linear regression

2.8 Summary of the Chapter

Linear Model,
$E(y \mid x) = f^T(x)\theta,\ Var(y \mid x) = \sigma^2,\ x \in \chi$ compact.
Select experimental conditions $x_1, \dots, x_n$ (*exact design*).
Observe the responses $y_1, \dots, y_n$.
Approximate design: Probability measure ζ.
The *information matrix*, $M(\zeta) = \int_\chi f(x)f^T(x)\zeta(dx)$, is generalized for an approximate design.
A *criterion function*, Φ, looks for some particular objective.
The *equivalence theorem* for approximate designs allows to check whether a particular design is optimal or not and provides a tool for developing algorithms.
D-optimality is the most popular criterion: Determinant of the information matrix.
Efficiency of a design:

$$\text{eff}_\Phi(\zeta) = \frac{\Phi[M(\zeta^*)]}{\Phi[M(\zeta)]}.$$

Table 2.3 shows a summary of the criteria with the corresponding efficiency bounds coming from the equivalence theorem. Tables 2.4, 2.5, 2.6, and 2.7 give well-known optimal designs for different criteria and typical models. Computing exact designs is a difficult task. Sometimes they depend on the prime factor decomposition of the sample size number. They “try to be” similar to the approximate designs, but this is not always the case.

Table 2.3 Summary of design criteria. Some complex efficiency bound is omitted

Criterion	Function	Efficiency bound	Meaning
D-	$\log\det M^{-1}(\xi)$ or $\det M^{-1/m}(\xi)$	$2-\frac{\max_x d(x,\xi)}{m}$, where $d(x,\xi)=f^T(x)M^{-1}(\xi)f(x)$ $\frac{m}{\max_x d(x,\xi)}$ (Atwood)	Ellipsoid volume
D_s-	$\log\det[M^{-1}(\xi)]_s$,		s parameters
L-	$\mathrm{tr}WM^{-}(\xi)$, W full rank matrix	$2-\frac{\max_x f^T(x)M^{-1}(\xi)WM^{-1}(\xi)f(x)}{\mathrm{tr}WM^{-1}(\xi)}$	linear combinations
A-	$\mathrm{tr}M^{-1}(\xi)$	$2-\frac{\max_x f^T(x)M^{-2}f(x)}{\mathrm{tr}M^{-1}(\xi)}$	Variances average ($H=I$ for L-optimality)
c-	$c^TM^{-}(\xi)c$	$2-\frac{\max_x f^T(x)M^{-}Parameterscc^TM^{-}(\xi)f(x)}{c^TM^{-}(\xi)c}$	One combination ($H=c$)
E-	λ_ξ^{-1}, minimum	$2-\frac{\max_x \sum_{i=1}^a \pi_i P_i^T f(x)f^T(x)P_i}{\lambda_{\min}[M(\xi)]}$, where $\lambda_{\min}[M(\xi)]P_i=M(\xi)P_i$, a the multiplicity of $\lambda_{\min}[M(\xi)]$, and $\sum_{i=1}^a \pi_i=1,\ 0\le\pi_i\le 1$	Maximum ellipsoid axis
MV-	$\max_i \left\{M^{-1}(\xi)\right\}_{ii}$		Maximum variance
G-	$\max_x f^T(x)M^{-1}(\xi)f(x)$		Prediction variance
I-	$\int_S f^T(x)M^{-1}(\xi)f(x)\mu(dx)$	Reduced to L-optimality	Mean prediction variance

Table 2.4 Some optimal designs for a few criteria for simple linear regression ($E(y|x) = \theta_0 + \theta_1 x$). Support points in the third and fourth columns and weights of the first point in the last column

Criterion	χ	Approximate OED	p
D- & G-	$[a, b]$	$a \quad b$	1/2
A-	$[a, b]$	$a \quad b$	$\frac{\sqrt{a^2+1}}{\sqrt{a^2+1}+\sqrt{b^2+1}}$
MV-	$[a, b]$	$a \quad b$	$1/2$ if $\lvert ab\rvert < 1 \,\&\, a^2+b^2 \le 2$, $\frac{\lvert b\rvert}{\lvert a\rvert+\lvert b\rvert}$ if $\lvert ab\rvert \ge 1$, $\frac{b^2-1}{b^2-a^2}$ if $\lvert ab\rvert < 1 \,\&\, a^2+b^2 > 2$

Table 2.5 Some optimal exact designs for a few criteria and simple linear regression. The sample size is denoted by n_e if it is even and n_o if it is odd

Criterion	χ	Exact OED
D-	$[a, b]$	$a(n_e/2, n_o/2, n_o/2+1) \quad b(n_e/2, n_o/2+1, n_o/2)$
G-	$[-1, 1]$	$-1(p) \quad 0(q) \quad 1(p), \quad q \in \{0, 1\},\ n = 2p + q$
A-	$[-b, b]$	$-b(n_e/2, n_o/2, n_o/2+1) \quad b(n_e/2, n_o/2+1, n_o/2)$, otherwise one in a middle point

Table 2.6 Some optimal designs for a few criteria and quadratic regression ($E(y|x) = \theta_0 + \theta_1 x + \theta_2 x^2$). Support points and weights between brackets

Criterion	χ	Approximate OED
D- & G-	$[a, b]$	$a(1/3) \quad \frac{(6+\sqrt{3})a-\sqrt{3}b}{6}(1/3) \quad b(1/3)$
A-	$[-1, 1]$	$-1(1/4) \quad 0(1/2) \quad 1(1/4)$

Table 2.7 Examples of optimal exact designs for a few cases and quadratic regression

Criterion	χ	Exact OED
D- & G-	$[-1, 1]$	$-1(n/3) \quad 0(n/3) \quad 1(n/3)$ if $n = \dot{3}$ More complex if $n \neq \dot{3}$
A-	$[-1, 1]$	$-1 \quad \alpha \quad 1$ (replicates as near as possible to $n/4,\ n/2,\ n/4$)

2.9 Exercises

Exercise 2.1 Consider a Gaussian polynomial model of degree m. Experiments are made at $m + 1$ values $x_0, \ldots, x_m$, of the explanatory variable. If the variance of any observation is constant, $\sigma^2(x) = \sigma^2$, prove that the determinant of the FIM is proportional to $(x_1 - x_0)^2(x_2 - x_1)^2(x_2 - x_0)^2 \cdots (x_m - x_0)^2$.

Exercise 2.2 Compute an A-optimal design for the model $y = \theta_0 + \theta_1 x + \theta_2 x^3 + \varepsilon,\ x \in \chi = [0, 1]$ using a similar procedure as in Example 2.9.

Solution

$$\begin{Bmatrix} 0 & 0.576 & 1 \\ 0.3288 & 0.4695 & 0.2016 \end{Bmatrix}.$$

Exercise 2.3 Compute c-optimal designs for $c_1 = (1, 0)^T$, $c_2 = (0, 1)^T$ for the model $y = \theta_0 \cos(x) + \theta_1 \sin(x) + \varepsilon$, $x \in \chi = [0, \pi/3]$ using the Elfving graphical procedure.

Solution

$$\xi_{c_1} = \begin{Bmatrix} 0 \\ 1 \end{Bmatrix}, \ \xi_{c_2} = \begin{Bmatrix} 0 & \pi/3 \\ 1/3 & 2/3 \end{Bmatrix}.$$

Exercise 2.4 (From Fedorov, 1972, p. 88) Prove that for a model

$$y = \theta_1 f_1(x) + \theta_2 f_2(x) + \varepsilon, \ x \in \chi = [a, b], \ a > 0$$

with symmetric variance $\sigma^2(x)$; f_1 even, that is $f_1(-x) = f_1(x)$, $x \in \chi$; and $f_2(x)$ odd, that is $f_2(-x) = -f_2(x)$, $x \in \chi$. If ξ^* is D-optimal then $M(\xi^*)$ is diagonal.

Solution Assume it is not diagonal and take $\tilde{\xi}$ a mirror image of ξ^*, that is, $\tilde{\xi}(x) = \xi^*(-x)$ for every $x \in \chi$. Then

$$\begin{aligned}
&\det M(\tilde{\xi}) \\
&= \det \begin{pmatrix} \sum_x \sigma^{-2}(x) f_1(-x)^2 \xi^*(x) & \sum_x \sigma^{-2}(-x) f_1(-x) f_2(-x) \xi^*(x) \\ \sum_x \sigma^{-2}(-x) f_1(-x) f_2(-x) \xi^*(x) & \sum_x \sigma^{-2}(x) f_2(-x)^2 \xi^*(x) \end{pmatrix} \\
&= \det \begin{pmatrix} \sum_x \sigma^{-2}(x) f_1(x)^2 \xi^*(x) & -\sum_x \sigma^{-2}(x) f_1(x) f_2(x) \xi^*(x) \\ -\sum_x \sigma^{-2}(x) f_1(x) f_2(x) \xi^*(x) & \sum_x \sigma^{-2}(x) f_2(x)^2 \xi^*(x) \end{pmatrix} \\
&= \det M(\xi^*),
\end{aligned}$$

although $M(\tilde{\xi}) \neq M(\xi^*)$. Since $-\log\det M(\xi)$ is strictly convex then

$$\begin{aligned}
-\log\det M\left[\frac{1}{2}M(\xi^*) + \frac{1}{2}M(\tilde{\xi})\right] &< -\left[\frac{1}{2}\log\det M(\xi^*) + \frac{1}{2}\log\det M(\tilde{\xi})\right] \\
&= -\log\det M(\xi^*)
\end{aligned}$$

meaning that $\frac{1}{2}M(\xi^*) + \frac{1}{2}M(\tilde{\xi})$ is better than the D-optimal design. Thus, $M(\xi^*)$ should be diagonal.

Chapter 3
Designing for Nonlinear Models

Once again, Box (1979): "Models, of course, are never true, but fortunately it is only necessary that they be useful."

3.1 What Is a Statistical Model? (Revisited)

Coming back to the first chapter (Sect. 1.1), a general model is being considered now. It may be called a nonlinear model since some of the conditions given in Sect. 2.1 for linear models fail. Let y be the response (univariate or multivariate) and assume x is a vector of explanatory variables. Assume the experiment is realized n times for n values $x_1, x_2, \ldots, x_n$ of x. Let $y_1, y_2, \ldots, y_n$ be the corresponding outcomes. A general parametric model trying to describe this relationship between both groups of variables is a parametric family of distributions defined by the pdfs:

$$\{h(y_1, y_2, \ldots, y_n \mid x_1, x_2, \ldots, x_n; \theta_1, \theta_2, \ldots, \theta_m) \mid \theta = (\theta_1, \theta_2, \ldots, \theta_m)^T \in \Theta\}.$$

An experimental condition x can be chosen on a compact *design space*, χ.

This definition includes all the parametric statistics such as t-tests, ANOVA, and any type of regression with any probability distribution, with correlated or uncorrelated observations. The later deserves particular treatment from the analysis and design point of view, and it will be considered in another chapter.

In a Bayesian approach the pdf $h(y_1, y_2, \ldots, y_n \mid x_1, x_2, \ldots, x_n; \theta_1, \theta_2, \ldots, \theta_m)$ may be understood as a conditional pdf given particular values of the parameters. Then the parameters will follow a prior marginal distribution completing the whole distribution of the model.

J. López-Fidalgo, *Optimal Experimental Design*, Lecture Notes in Statistics 226,
https://doi.org/10.1007/978-3-031-35918-7_3

3.2 Uncorrelated Observations

If the observations are uncorrelated, the joint distribution is the product of the marginal distributions, usually assumed identical except for the different values of x. Then the model can be thought as a family of univariate distributions for each observation y from an experiment realized at x:

$$\{h(y|x; \theta_1, \theta_2, \ldots, \theta_m) \,|\, \theta = (\theta_1, \theta_2, \ldots, \theta_m)^T \in \Theta\}.$$

Assuming $\mathrm{E}(y \mid x) = \eta(x, \theta)$, $Var(y \mid x) = \sigma^2$ the model is usually represented as a typical regression model

$$y = \eta(x, \theta) + \varepsilon,$$

where ε is a random variable with mean zero and constant variance σ^2.

Example 3.1 Some particular nonlinear models on the parameters of the mean $\eta(x, \theta)$:

1. Exponential: $\theta_1 e^{-\theta_2 x}$.
2. Michaelis–Menten: $\frac{\theta_1 x}{\theta_2 + x}$.
3. Trigonometric: $\theta_1 \cos(\theta_2 x) + \theta_3 \cos(\theta_4 x)$.
4. Gompertz: $\theta_1 e^{-e^{\theta_2 - \theta_3 x}}$.

In these cases there is lack of linearity on some of the parameters in the mean. Thus, they are nonlinear models with any kind of distribution, in particular under normality.

3.3 Fisher Information

The *Fisher Information Matrix* for a particular experimental condition x is:

$$I(x, \theta) = \mathrm{E}_h \left[\left(\frac{\partial \ell(x, \theta)}{\partial \theta} \right) \left(\frac{\partial \ell(x, \theta)}{\partial \theta^T} \right) \right] = -\mathrm{E}_h \left[\left(\frac{\partial^2 \ell(x, \theta)}{\partial \theta^2} \right) \right]. \tag{3.1}$$

The expectation E_h is computed here with respect to the distribution with pdf $h(y|x; \theta)$ and $\ell(x, \theta)$ is the log-likelihood for this sample distribution. The last inequality holds under basic regularity conditions. This matrix is a measure of the information provided by x to the estimation of the model.

For general nonlinear models the FIM might not be of the form $I(x, \theta) = f^T(x, \theta) f(x, \theta)$ for some function f. The exponential family guarantees the existence of this function as it will be seen in the next sections. Additionally, some distributions of the response may not allow the closed-form computation of the expectation. This happens, for instance, for a mixture of normal distributions (see Sect. 6.2 for an example).

For an approximate design

$$\xi = \begin{Bmatrix} x_1 \cdots x_k \\ p_1 \cdots p_k \end{Bmatrix}$$

the associated FIM will be

$$M(\xi, \theta) = \sum_{x \in \chi} \xi(x) I(x, \theta).$$

The inverse of the FIM is asymptotically proportional to the covariance matrix of the MLEs of the parameters (see Appendix B).

Some problems and restrictions arise for nonlinear models. On the one hand, the FIM depends on the parameters to be estimated. Some solutions for this can be implemented:

- *Locally Φ-optimal designs* (Chernoff, 1953): This means giving nominal values to the parameters, say $\theta^{(0)}$, as a guess and computing the optimal design, $\xi_{\theta^{(0)}}$, for those values. Thus, an error is introduced in this computation of the true optimal design, $\xi^\star$, with respect to the unknown true values of the parameters, say $\theta^\star$. For locally optimal designs a sensitivity analysis checking relative efficiencies in a neighborhood of the nominal values of the parameters is highly recommended.
- *Minimax designs:* The criterion is modified here to minimize the worst choice of the parameters. A typical formulation is (Atkinson & Fedorov, 1988)

$$\min_{\xi \in \Xi} \max_{\theta} \Phi[M(\xi, \theta)].$$

- *Sequential designs:* The design is obtained in several steps taking into account the observations in the previous step to estimate the parameters and use that for designing in the next step. They are also called adaptive designs. Box and Hunter (1965) introduced sequential designs for the first time and Fedorov and Pázman (1968) gave an adaptive Bayesian procedure for simultaneous model discrimination and parameter estimation. Then the first edition of Chernoff (2000) in 1972 made an extensive introduction to this type of experiments.
- *Bayesian designs:* Instead of risking assuming a particular choice of the nominal values of the parameters, a prior distribution, $\pi(\theta)$, can be considered. A simple pseudo-Bayesian formulation may be

$$\min_{\xi \in \Xi} \mathrm{E}_\pi\{\Phi[M(\xi, \theta)]\}.$$

The expectation is computed with the prior distribution. This is a Bayesian approach to compute optimal designs for computing MLEs. A pure Bayesian point of view should consider optimal designs for computing Bayesian estimators (Chaloner & Verdinelli, 1995). This will be considered in (Chap. 4. Pilz, 1993) offers a good introduction to Bayesian designs.

On the other hand, enough sample size is needed for a good approximation. Thus, if the sample size is small more justification is needed, for example, doing some simulation. For this we do not need strictly a good approximation. It will be enough if the specific criterion runs monotonically with both matrices, the inverse of the FIM and the covariance matrix of the estimators.

Remark 3.1 D-optimality is invariant by reparameterization of the model under any of the versions of the exponential family. Let $g(\tau) = \theta$ be a one-to-one reparameterization with g continuously differentiable. Thus,

$$\frac{\partial \eta}{\partial \tau} = \frac{\partial g}{\partial \tau}\left(\frac{\partial \eta}{\partial \theta}\right)_{\theta=g(\tau)}.$$

Assuming constant variance for simplicity, without loss of generality, the information matrix for the vector of parameters τ is then proportional to

$$I_\tau(x,\tau) = \frac{\partial g}{\partial \tau}\left(\frac{\partial \eta}{\partial \theta}\right)_{\theta=g(\tau)}\left(\frac{\partial \eta}{\partial \theta^T}\right)_{\theta=g(\tau)}\frac{\partial g}{\partial \tau^T} = \frac{\partial g}{\partial \tau} I_\theta(x,\theta)\frac{\partial g}{\partial \tau^T},$$

where I_θ and I_τ stand for the FIM of the models corresponding to those parameters. Therefore,

$$M_\tau(x,\tau) = \frac{\partial g}{\partial \tau} M_\theta(x,\theta)\frac{\partial g}{\partial \tau^T}$$

and the determinant is

$$\det M_\tau(\xi) = \det\left(\frac{\partial g}{\partial \tau}\right)^2 \det M_\theta(x,\theta),$$

where

$$\det\left(\frac{\partial g}{\partial \tau}\right)^2$$

does not depend on the design.

This is an exclusive property of D-optimality. The matrix $\frac{\partial g}{\partial \tau}$ changes the criterion for the other given in this book. For linear criteria, for instance, this matrix changes the matrix with the coefficients,

$$\operatorname{tr}\left(W\frac{\partial g}{\partial \tau}\right) M_\theta^{-1}(x,\theta)\left(\frac{\partial g}{\partial \tau^T}A^T\right) = \operatorname{tr}\left[\left(\frac{\partial g}{\partial \tau^T}A^T W\frac{\partial g}{\partial \tau}\right) M_\theta^{-1}(x,\theta)\right]$$
$$= \operatorname{tr}\left(W' M_\theta^{-1}(x,\theta)\right),$$

and the directional derivative can be computed easily through the new matrix W'.

3.4 Equivalence Theorem for Nonlinear Models

The usual equivalence theorem applies here straightforward (see, e.g., White, 1973).

Theorem 3.1 *Let Φ be a convex criterion, then $\xi^\star$ is Φ-optimal if and only if*

$$\partial\Phi[M(\xi^\star,\theta), M(\xi,\theta)] \geq 0,$$

for any approximate design ξ.

If Φ is differentiable the optimality condition can be relaxed to $\psi(x,\xi^*,\theta) \geq 0,\ x \in \chi$, where

$$\psi(x,\xi,\theta) = \partial\Phi[M(\xi,\theta), I(x,\theta)]$$
$$= \operatorname{tr}\{\nabla\Phi[M(\xi,\theta)][I(x,\theta) - M(\xi,\theta)]\}$$

is the so-called sensitivity function.

3.5 Natural Exponential Family

For linear models the FIM at a particular point x is proportional to $f(x,\theta)f^T(x,\theta)$, where $f(x,\theta)$ is the vector of regressors, the "coefficients" of the parameters. In this and next sections, sufficient conditions will be studied when the FIM for nonlinear models is of this type. Thus, it is equivalent to a linear model in terms of OED.

A popular family of distributions is the so-called *exponential family*. A typical definition is used for generalized linear models (GLMs) defined by a pdf of the type

$$h(y|\beta) = \exp\left[\frac{\beta y - b(\beta)}{a(\phi)} + c(y,\phi)\right],$$

where ϕ is a *scale parameter* and β is the *natural parameter*. We will refer to it as the *natural exponential family*. For that the log-likelihood is computed:

$$\ell(\beta) = \frac{\beta y - b(\beta)}{a(\phi)} + c(y, \phi).$$

Since

$$\frac{\partial \ell(\beta)}{\partial \beta} = \frac{y - b'(\beta)}{a(\phi)}$$

and

$$\begin{aligned} \mathrm{E}\left(\frac{\partial \ell(\beta)}{\partial \beta}\right) &= \int \frac{\partial \log h(y|\beta)}{\partial \beta} h(y|\beta) dy = \int \frac{\partial h(y|\beta)}{\partial \beta} dy \\ &= \frac{\partial \int h(y|\beta) dy}{\partial \beta} = \frac{\partial 1}{\partial \beta} = 0, \end{aligned}$$

then

$$\mathrm{E}(y) = b'(\beta).$$

Since

$$\frac{\partial^2 \ell(\beta)}{\partial \beta^2} = \frac{-b''(\beta)}{a(\phi)}$$

and again exchanging the derivatives with the integral of the expectation

$$\begin{aligned} \mathrm{E}\left(\frac{\partial^2 \ell(\beta)}{\partial \beta^2}\right) &= \int \frac{\partial^2 \log h(y|\beta)}{\partial \beta^2} h(y|\beta) dy \\ &= \int \frac{\frac{\partial^2 h(y|\beta)}{\partial \beta^2} h(y|\beta) - \frac{\partial h(y|\beta)}{\partial \beta} \frac{\partial h(y|\beta)}{\partial \beta^T}}{h(y|\beta)^2} h(y|\beta) dy \\ &= \int \frac{\partial^2 h(y|\beta)}{\partial \beta^2} dy - \int \frac{\frac{\partial h(y|\beta)}{\partial \beta}}{h(y|\beta)} \frac{\frac{\partial h(y|\beta)}{\partial \beta^T}}{h(y|\beta)} h(y|\beta) dy \\ &= \frac{\partial^2}{\partial \beta^2} \int h(y|\beta) dy - \int \frac{\partial \log h(y|\beta)}{\partial \beta} \frac{\partial \log h(y|\beta)}{\partial \beta^T} h(y|\beta) dy \\ &= -\mathrm{E}\left(\frac{\partial \ell(\beta)}{\partial \beta} \frac{\partial \ell(\beta)}{\partial \beta^T}\right), \end{aligned}$$

then

$$\mathrm{var}(y) = b''(\beta)a(\phi).$$

Now a vector of explanatory variables, x, is introduced modeling the natural parameter,

$$\beta = \eta(x, \theta)$$

and assuming ϕ is known. Then

$$h(y|x, \theta) = \exp\left\{\frac{\eta(x, \theta)y - b[\eta(x, \theta)]}{a(\phi)} + c(y, \phi)\right\}$$

and the log-likelihood is then

$$\ell(\theta) = \frac{\eta(x, \theta)y - b[\eta(x, \theta)]}{a(\phi)} + c(y, \phi).$$

After deriving twice

$$\frac{\partial \ell(\theta)}{\partial \theta} = \frac{\{y - b'[\eta(x, \theta)]\}}{a(\phi)} \frac{\partial \eta(x, \theta)}{\partial \theta},$$

$$\frac{\partial^2 \ell(\theta)}{\partial \theta^2} = \frac{\{y - b'[\eta(x, \theta)]\} \frac{\partial^2 \eta(x,\theta)}{\partial \theta^2} - b''[\eta(x, \theta)] \frac{\partial \eta(x,\theta)}{\partial \theta} \frac{\partial \eta(x,\theta)}{\partial \theta^T}}{a(\phi)},$$

the FIM is

$$I(x, \theta) = -\mathrm{E}\left[\frac{\partial^2 \ell(\theta)}{\partial \theta^2}\right] = \frac{b''[\eta(x, \theta)]}{a(\phi)} \frac{\partial \eta(x, \theta)}{\partial \theta} \frac{\partial \eta(x, \theta)}{\partial \theta^T}.$$

Defining $f(x, \theta) = \sqrt{\frac{b''[\eta(x,\theta)]}{a(\phi)}} \frac{\partial \eta(x,\theta)}{\partial \theta}$ the FIM is of the type mentioned above. In particular, this is the FIM of any of the following models:

$$y = b''[\eta(x, \theta^{(0)})] \frac{\partial \eta(x, \theta^{(0)})}{\partial \theta^T} \theta + \varepsilon, \ \mathrm{var}(\varepsilon) = b''[\eta(x, \theta^{(0)})] a(\phi) \quad (3.2)$$

or

$$y = \sqrt{\frac{b''[\eta(x, \theta^{(0)})]}{a(\phi)}} \frac{\partial \eta(x, \theta^{(0)})}{\partial \theta^T} \theta + \varepsilon, \ \mathrm{var}(\varepsilon) = 1. \quad (3.3)$$

for some specific nominal values of the parameters $\theta^{(0)}$.

Let us consider now the original model in the traditional form:

$$y = b'[\eta(x,\theta)] + \varepsilon, \ \operatorname{var}(y) = b''[\eta(x,\theta)]a(\phi). \tag{3.4}$$

After a first-order Taylor approximation of the mean around a nominal value of the parameter $\theta^{(0)}$,

$$b'[\eta(x,\theta)] \approx b'[\eta(x,\theta^{(0)})] + \frac{\partial b'[\eta(x,\theta^{(0)})]}{\partial\theta^T}(\theta - \theta^{(0)}).$$

Redefining

$$\tilde{y} = y - b'[\eta(x,\theta^{(0)})] + \frac{\partial b'[\eta(x,\theta^{(0)})]}{\partial\theta^T}\theta^{(0)},$$

then an equivalent approximated model will be:

$$\tilde{y} = \frac{\partial b'[\eta(x,\theta^{(0)})]}{\partial\theta^T}\theta + \varepsilon, \ \operatorname{var}(\tilde{y}) = b''[\eta(x,\theta^{(0)})]a(\phi).$$

But

$$\frac{\partial b'[\eta(x,\theta)]}{\partial\theta} = \frac{\partial\eta(x,\theta)}{\partial\theta}b''[\eta(x,\theta)].$$

Thus, the resulting model is of type (3.2). And dividing by the square root of the variance a model of type (3.3) is obtained. Therefore, the following theorem may be stated.

Theorem 3.2 *Let a model be defined through the natural exponential family*

$$h(y|x,\theta) = \exp\left\{\frac{\eta(x,\theta)y - b[\eta(x,\theta)]}{a(\phi)} + c(y,\phi)\right\},$$

assuming ϕ is known. Then its FIM is the same as the information matrix of the linearized models (3.2) and (3.3).

Remark 3.2 Under the conditions above if the mean is directly modeled by $b'(\beta) = \mu(x,\theta)$ and β can be worked out, $\beta = \eta(x,\theta)$, then the theorem applies here directly.

Remark 3.3 In the result summarized in the theorem, the original model (3.4) is linearized in two steps:

1. The mean is linearized and the variance approximated directly at the nominal values of the parameters.
2. The mean is divided by the standard deviation.

Another approximation can be done in a different way:

1. The mean is divided by the standard deviation.
2. The new mean is linearized around the nominal values of the parameters.

Acting in this way, that is, deriving

$$\frac{b'[\eta(x,\theta)]}{\sqrt{b''[\eta(x,\theta)]}},$$

the approximated model will be

$$y = \left\{\sqrt{b''[\eta(x,\theta^{(0)})]} - \frac{b'[\eta(x,\theta^{(0)})]b'''[\eta(x,\theta^{(0)})]}{b''[\eta(x,\theta^{(0)})]\sqrt{b''[\eta(x,\theta^{(0)})]}}\right\}$$
$$\times \frac{1}{\sqrt{a(\phi)}}\frac{\partial\eta(x,\theta^{(0)})}{\partial\theta^T}\theta + \varepsilon, \ \mathrm{var}(\varepsilon) = 1.$$

This approximation does not match the Cramer–Rao theorem for the FIM. The difference is in the term

$$\frac{b'[\eta(x,\theta^{(0)})]b'''[\eta(x,\theta^{(0)})]}{b''[\eta(x,\theta^{(0)})]\sqrt{b''[\eta(x,\theta^{(0)})]}},$$

which needs to be explored in more detail. In particular, if the third derivative of b vanishes at the nominal value, then both approaches are equivalent.

Remark 3.4 A *generalized linear model* is considered as a particular case of the natural exponential family. The distributions considered now are given by

$$h(y|\beta) = \exp\left[\frac{\beta y - b(\beta)}{a(\phi)} + c(y,\phi)\right],$$

where $\mu = \mathrm{E}(y) = b'(\beta)$ is the so-called *location parameter* and $g(\mu) = f^T(x)\theta$ is the *link function* with $\beta = \eta[f^T(x)\theta]$. Usually $a(\phi) = \phi$ is assumed known.

The MLEs follow asymptotically a normal distribution $\mathcal{N}(\theta, (X^T W X)^{-1}\phi)$ with $W = \mathrm{diag}\{b''[\eta(f^T(x)\theta)]^{-1}g'(\mu)^{-2}\}$.

3.6 General Exponential Family

In the literature there is another typical definition of the exponential family. It is the so-called *general exponential family*:

$$h(y|\beta) = \exp[A(\beta)B(y) + C(y) + D(\beta)],$$

where $A(\beta)$ and $B(y)$ can be vector functions, $C(y)$ and $D(\beta)$ are scalar functions, and β is a vector of parameters. The natural exponential family may be considered as a special case for $A(\beta) = \beta$, $B(y) = y$ if parameter ϕ is included in the pdf. Examples are the Binomial, Gamma, Inverse Gaussian, Negative Binomial, Normal, or Poisson distributions. The log-normal distribution is in the general exponential family, but not in the natural exponential family. In what follows $A(\beta)$, $B(y)$ and β will be considered as scalars. This is to make keep an easier notation, although the results can be generalized straightforward.

These are typical computations for the general exponential family:

$$\mathrm{E}[B(y)] = \frac{-D'(\beta)}{A'(\beta)},$$

$$\mathrm{var}[B(y)] = \frac{A''(\beta)D'(\beta) - A'(\beta)D''(\beta)}{A'(\beta)^3}.$$

Modeling the parameter $\beta = \eta(x, \theta)$, then

$$\frac{\partial \ell(\theta)}{\partial \theta} = \{A'[\eta(x,\theta)]B(y) - D'[\eta(x,\theta)]\}\frac{\partial \eta(x,\theta)}{\partial \theta},$$

and the FIM is then

$$\begin{aligned} I(x,\theta) &= \mathrm{E}\left[\frac{\partial \ell(\theta)}{\partial \theta}\frac{\partial \ell(\theta)}{\partial \theta^T}\right] \\ &= \frac{\mathrm{var}[B(y)]}{A'[\eta(x,\theta)]^2}\frac{\partial \eta(x,\theta)}{\partial \theta}\frac{\partial \eta(x,\theta)}{\partial \theta^T}. \end{aligned}$$

Calling again

$$f(x) = \sqrt{\frac{\mathrm{var}[B(y)]}{A'[\eta(x,\theta)]^2}}\frac{\partial \eta(x,\theta)}{\partial \theta}.$$

The traditional linearized model is obtained.

Thus, the practical procedure to compute the FIM for this family is as follows:

1. Consider the exponential family distribution modeling: $\mathrm{E}(y) = \eta(x,\theta)$, $\mathrm{var}(y) = \sigma^2$.
2. Perform the Taylor expansion around $\theta^{(0)}$:

$$\eta(x,\theta) \approx \eta(x,\theta^{(0)}) + \sum_{i=1}^{m}\left(\frac{\partial \eta(x,\theta)}{\partial \theta_i}\right)_{\theta^{(0)}}(\theta_i - \theta_i^{(0)}).$$

3. Approximate the mean to an equivalent linear model with $\tilde{f}_i(x) = \left(\frac{\partial\eta(x,\theta)}{\partial\theta_i}\right)_{\theta^{(0)}}; i = 1, \ldots, m,$

$$\mathrm{E}(y) = \sum_{i=1}^{m} \tilde{f}_i(x)\theta_i.$$

Example 3.2 Three families of probability distribution models coming from an example given by Tommasi et al. (2016) are trying to model the same phenomenon, all in the same design space $\chi = [a, b]$,

1. Weibull distribution:

$$h_1(y; \omega, \eta) = \frac{\omega}{\eta}\left(\frac{y}{\eta}\right)^{\omega-1} \exp\left[-\left(\frac{y}{\eta}\right)^{\omega}\right],$$

where parameter η is modeled by $\eta = \theta_1 \exp\left(\frac{-\theta_2}{x}\right)$. As a consequence, the mean lifetime is proportional to the Arrhenius model, that is,
$\mathrm{E}_{h_1}(y) = \Gamma\left(\frac{1}{\omega} + 1\right)\theta_1 \exp\left(\frac{-\theta_2}{x}\right)$.
2. Gamma distribution:

$$h_2(y; \nu, \phi) = \frac{y^{\nu-1}}{\phi^{\nu}\Gamma(\nu)} \exp\left(-\frac{y}{\phi}\right),$$

where $\phi = \theta_1 \exp\left(\frac{-\theta_2}{x}\right)$. Then the mean lifetime is proportional to the Arrhenius model once more, that is, $\mathrm{E}_{h_2}(Y) = \nu\,\theta_1 \exp\left(\frac{-\theta_2}{x}\right)$.
3. Log-normal distribution:

$$h_3(y; \mu, \sigma) = \frac{1}{\sqrt{2\pi}\sigma y} \exp\left[-\frac{(\log y - \mu)^2}{2\sigma^2}\right],$$

where $\mathrm{Median}(y) = e^{\mu} = C_L \exp\left(\frac{B_L}{x}\right)$, hence $\mu = \log\theta - 1 + \frac{\theta_2}{x}$. Thus, the mean lifetime is proportional to the Arrhenius model again, that is, $\mathrm{E}_{h_3}(y) = \exp\left(\frac{\sigma^2}{2}\right)\theta_1 \exp\left(\frac{-\theta_2}{x}\right)$.

A more elegant generalization of the three distribution is the generalized gamma distribution (Stacy, 1962), which includes as particular cases the three distributions considered in this example. The pdf of this distribution is

$$h(y; a, p, d) = \frac{p}{\Gamma(\frac{d}{p})a^d} y^{d-1} e^{-\left(\frac{y}{a}\right)^p}, \quad y \geq 0,$$

and for the following values of the parameters, we obtain the three previous models:

1. Weibull distribution: $p = d = \omega,\ a = \eta$.
2. Gamma distribution: $p = 1,\ d = \nu,\ a = \phi$.
3. Log-normal distribution: $p = \lambda/\sigma, d = \frac{1}{\lambda\sigma}, a = e^{\mu + \frac{2\sigma}{\lambda}\log(\lambda)}$, then $\lambda \to 0$.

The generalized gamma distribution is within the general exponential family, and the derivation of the FIM for the model $a = \eta(x, \theta) = \theta_1 e^{-\theta_2/x}$ becomes very friendly after some algebra. The log-likelihood is

$$\ell(\theta) = \log p - \log\Gamma(d/p) - d\log[\theta_1 e^{-\theta_2/x}] + (d-1)\log y - \frac{y^p}{\left(\theta_1 e^{-\theta_2/x}\right)^p}.$$

After differentiating twice, computing the expectation taking into account that for this distribution $\mathrm{E}(y^p) = \frac{d}{p}a$, then the FIM at one point, $M(\xi_x, \theta)$, is proportional to

$$\begin{pmatrix} 1/\theta_1^2 & -1/\theta_1 x \\ -1/\theta_1 x & 1/x^2 \end{pmatrix}.$$

Thus, the linear model associate has the vector of regressors $f^T(x) = (1, 1/x^2)$. It becomes simple linear regression for the design space $\chi = [1/b, 1/a]$.

3.7 Sensitivity Analysis

Since nominal values of the parameters are needed in advance for the computation of the optimal design, a sensitivity analysis will help to measure the robustness of the optimal design with respect to possible true values of the parameters.

Assuming M_θ is the information matrix computed with the values of the parameters θ, the relative efficiency is defined as:

$$\mathrm{eff}_{\theta^\star}(\xi_{\theta^{(0)}}) = \frac{\Phi[M_{\theta^\star}(\xi^\star)]}{\Phi[M_{\theta^\star}(\xi_{\theta^{(0)}})]}.$$

If explicit designs can be found depending on general possible true values of the parameters, the sensitivity analysis can be very informative. Usually, a figure or a table with carefully chosen potential true values gives the practitioner a clue for the risk of a wrong choice of the nominal values.

3.8 Illustrative Example

The example considered now shows how to compute optimal designs without an algorithm making some assumptions at the beginning and checking whether the equivalence theorem holds for the design computed. In other words, a restricted optimal design is computed within a simple class of designs where we guess the actual design remains. Then we check that this design is actually optimal with the GET.

Let y be a normally distributed r.v. with constant variance and mean:

$$E(y) = \alpha_1 e^{\beta_1 x} + \cdots + \alpha_m e^{\beta_m x}, \, x \in \chi = [0, 1].$$

This is the typical compartmental model describing a system with a number of compartments with possible flow between them at specific rates. Optimal designs for this type of models have been studied widely in the literature, for example, by Dette et al. (2006), Biedermann et al. (2007), Amo-Salas et al. (2012).

The FIM for this model is the same as the information matrix for the linear model given by

$$f_i(x) = \left(\frac{\partial \eta}{\partial \alpha_i} \right)_{(\alpha^{(0)}, \beta^{(0)})} = e^{\beta_i^{(0)} x}$$

and

$$g_i(x) = \left(\frac{\partial \eta}{\partial \beta_i} \right)_{(\alpha^{(0)}, \beta^{(0)})} = \alpha_i^{(0)} x e^{\beta_i^{(0)} x}.$$

Thus, the final model is then

$$\begin{aligned} E(y) &= \alpha^t f(x) + \beta^t g(x) \\ &= \alpha_1 e^{\beta_1^{(0)} x} + \cdots + \alpha_m e^{\beta_m^{(0)} x} + \beta_1 \alpha_1^{(0)} x e^{\beta_1^{(0)} x} + \cdots + \beta_m \alpha_m^{(0)} x e^{\beta_m^{(0)} x}. \end{aligned}$$

The FIM for $m = 2$ is

$$I(x, \theta) = \begin{pmatrix} e^{2\beta_1 x} & e^{\beta_1 x + \beta_2 x} & \alpha_1 e^{2\beta_1 x} & \alpha_2 e^{\beta_1 x + \beta_2 x} \\ e^{\beta_1 x + \beta_2 x} & e^{2\beta_2 x} & \alpha_1 e^{\beta_1 x + \beta_2 x} & \alpha_2 e^{2\beta_2 x} \\ \alpha_1 e^{2\beta_1 x} & \alpha_1 e^{\beta_1 x + \beta_2 x} & \alpha_1^2 e^{2\beta_1 x} & \alpha_1 \alpha_2 e^{\beta_1 x + \beta_2 x} \\ \alpha_2 e^{\beta_1 x + \beta_2 x} & \alpha_2 e^{2\beta_2 x} & \alpha_1 \alpha_2 e^{\beta_1 x + \beta_2 x} & \alpha_2^2 e^{2\beta_2 x} \end{pmatrix},$$

for $\theta = (\alpha_1, \ldots, \alpha_m, \beta_1, \ldots, \beta_m)^T$ and the determinant for a general four-point design, with points x_1, x_2, x_3, x_4 and weights p_1, p_2, p_3, p_4 is

$$\begin{aligned}\alpha_1^2\alpha_2^2 p_1 p_2 p_3 p_4 \Big[&(x_1 - x_4)(x_2 - x_3)e^{\beta_1(x_1+x_4)+\beta_2(x_2+x_3)} \\ &+(x_1 - x_4)(x_2 - x_3)e^{\beta_1(x_2+x_3)+\beta_2(x_1+x_4)} \\ &-(x_1 - x_3)(x_2 - x_4)e^{\beta_1(x_2+x_4)+\beta_2(x_1+x_3)} \\ &-(x_1 - x_3)(x_2 - x_4)e^{\beta_1(x_1+x_3)+\beta_2(x_2+x_4)} \\ &+(x_1 - x_2)(x_3 - x_4)e^{\beta_1(x_3+x_4)+\beta_2(x_1+x_2)} \\ &+(x_1 - x_2)(x_3 - x_4)e^{\beta_1(x_1+x_2)+\beta_2(x_3+x_4)}\Big]^2.\end{aligned}$$

This shows that if the optimal design has four points, it does not depend on α_1 and α_2, and the optimal weights must be equal:

$$\xi = \left\{ \begin{array}{cccc} x_1 & x_2 & x_3 & x_4 \\ 1/4 & 1/4 & 1/4 & 1/4 \end{array} \right\}. \tag{3.5}$$

Assuming as nominal values $\beta_1 = 1$ and $\beta_2 = -1$ and taking $x_1 = 0, x_4 = 1$, the determinant is now proportional to:

$$\begin{aligned}e^{-2(x_3+x_4+1)} \Big(&e^{2(x_3+x_4)}(x_3 - x_4) + e^2(x_3 - x_4) + e^{2x_3}x_3(x_4 - 1) \\ &+x_3 e^{2x_4+2}(x_4 - 1) - e^{2x_3+2}(x_3 - 1)x_4 - (x_3 - 1)e^{2x_4}x_4\Big)^2.\end{aligned}$$

Figure 3.1 shows the determinant of the FIM for designs of type (3.5). The maximum is reached at $x_2 = 0.274$, $x_3 = 0.726$. Figure 3.2 displays the sensi-

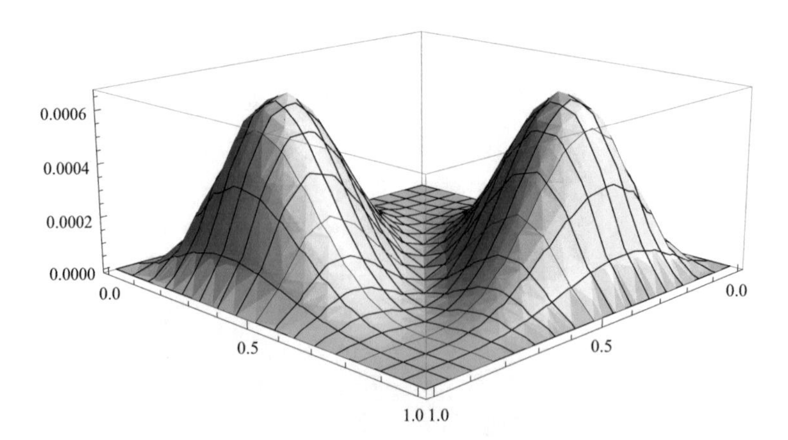

Fig. 3.1 Determinant of the FIM for designs of type (3.5) with $x_1 = 0$ and $x_2 = 1$

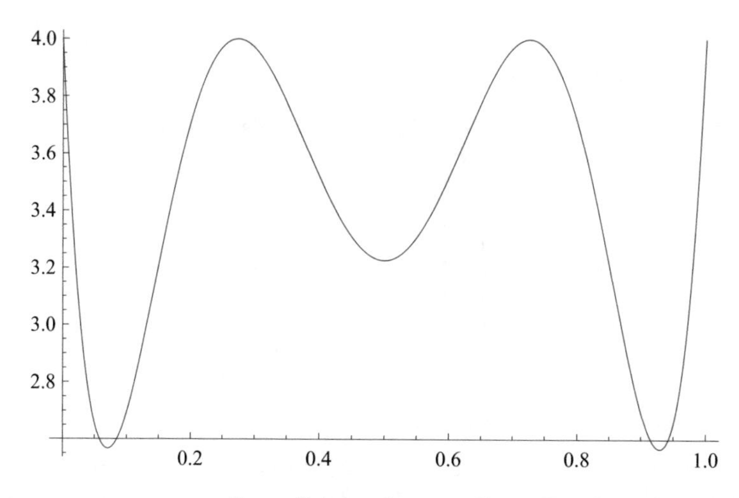

Fig. 3.2 Sensitivity function $(f^T(x), g^T(x))M^{-1}(\xi^\star, \theta)(f^T(x), g^T(x))^T$ for the best design of type (3.5)

tivity function of this design $(f^T(x), g^T(x))M^{-1}(\xi^\star, \theta)(f^T(x), g^T(x))^T$, which is (numerically) below 4, the number of parameters. This means the design computed with the assumptions made (four-point design with extreme values 0 and 1) is actually D-optimal among all possible designs in the space $\chi = [0, 1]$.

3.9 Polynomial Models and Chebyshev systems

The theory of *Chebyshev systems* and *orthogonal polynomials* provides interesting results for finding optimal designs or determining their number of support points for differentiable criteria by using the GET. It is said that $r+1$ linearly independent real-valued continuous functions, $\{g_0, \ldots, g_r\}$, defined on a compact set $\chi = [a, b]$, forms a Chebyshev system if every nontrivial linear combination of the $r+1$ functions, say $a_0 g_0(x) + \cdots + a_r g_r(x)$ with $\sum_{i=0}^r a_i^2 > 0$, has at most $r+1$ zeros, counting multiplicity. Checking this property directly is not easy in general, but there is an equivalent definition (Karlin & Studden, 1966, Theorem 4.1). Celant and Broniatowski (2017) is a good recent reference for the application of Chebyshev systems to optimal experimental designs.

Theorem 3.3 *A Chebyshev system, $\{g_0, \ldots, g_r\}$, satisfies the necessary and sufficient condition that the determinant of the matrix*

$$\begin{pmatrix} g_0(x_0) & \cdots & g_r(x_0) \\ \cdots & \cdots & \cdots \\ g_0(x_r) & \cdots & g_r(x_r) \end{pmatrix}$$

has the same sign for any $x_0 < \cdots < x_r$ in χ.

This is still not easy to check in most of the cases and there is a much easier way of checking whether a system is Chebyshev or not.

Theorem 3.4 *A Chebyshev system, $\{g_0, \ldots, g_r\}$, satisfies the necessary a sufficient condition that the Wronskian matrix of the system*

$$\begin{pmatrix} g_0(x) & \cdots & g_r(x) \\ g_0'(x) & \cdots & g_r'(x) \\ g_0''(x) & \cdots & g_r''(x) \\ \cdots & \cdots & \cdots \\ g_0^{(r)}(x) & \cdots & g_r^{(r)}(x) \end{pmatrix}$$

has positive determinant for all $x \in \chi$.

From the GET the sensitivity function must satisfy $\psi(x, \xi^\star) \leq 0$ for all $x \in \chi$ for an optimal design $\xi^\star$ with equality at the support points. Sometimes the sensitivity function and its derivative are linear combinations of several functions that form a Chebyshev system on χ. Using the reasoning in an inverse way, if the Wronskian property is satisfied for those functions, then the number of zeroes of the linear combinations defining the sensitivity function and its derivative is bounded by a known number. This can be used to study the support points of the optimal design.

A particular and very successful example of application is D-optimality for polynomial models. In what follows let a polynomial model be $\mathrm{E}(y) = \theta_0 + \theta_1 x + \theta_2 x^2 + \cdots + \theta_{m-1} x^{m-1}$ with $\mathrm{var}(y) = \sigma^2(x) = \lambda(x)$, $x \in \chi$, where χ is an interval with extremes a and b. Karlin and Studden (1966) provided the following result.

Theorem 3.5 *There is a D-optimal design ξ^* with m points in its support if one of the following conditions is satisfied:*

(i) $\{1, \lambda(x), \lambda(x)x, \lambda(x)x^2, \ldots, \lambda(x)x^{2(m-1)}\}$ *is a Chebyshev system.*
(ii) $\lambda(x) = P^{-1}(x)$, *where* $P(x) > 0$ *is a polynomial in* $[a, b]$ *and* $P^{(2m-1)}(x) \neq 0$ *for* $x \in (a, b)$.
(iii) $\lambda(x) = P^{-1}(x)$, *where* $P(x) > 0$ *is a polynomial in* $[a, b]$ *with degree less than or equal to* $2m - 1$.
(iv) $\lambda(x)$ *can be approximated uniformly by functions of type (iii).*

Proof Let ξ be an approximate design supported at m points, then

$$\det M(\xi) = \prod_{k=0}^{m-1} \xi(x_k)\sigma^{-2}(x_i) \left| \prod_{i<j}^{m-1} (x_i - x_j) \right| .$$

If it is optimal then the weights have to be equal, $\xi(x_i) = 1/m,\ i = 0, \ldots, m-1$ and the sensitivity function nonnegative,

$$\psi(x, \xi) = m - \sigma^{-2}(x) f^T(x) M^{-1}(\xi) f(x) \geq 0,\ x \in \chi.$$

The equality, $\psi(x, \xi) = 0$, is reached at the support points, that is,

$$m\sigma^2(x) - f^T(x)M^{-1}(\xi)f(x) = 0.$$

If it has at least $m+1$ zeroes, then $\psi(x, \xi) - \gamma$ has at least $2m$ zeroes for some $\gamma > 0$, say $a \leq x_1 < \cdots < x_{2m} \leq b$, and taking into account that $f^T(x)M^{-1}(\xi)f(x)$ is a polynomial of degree $2(m-1)$, then there is a system of equations of the type

$$\sigma^2(x_j)a_0 + \sum_{i=0}^{2m-1} a_i x_j^{i-1} = 0,\ j = 1, \ldots, 2m.$$

(i) The Chebyshev system property states that the only solutions have to be $a_0 = a_1 = \cdots = a_{2m-1} = 0$ and therefore

$$q(x) = (m - \gamma)\sigma^2(x) - f^T(x)M^{-1}(\xi)f(x)$$

has at most $2m - 1$ zeroes in $[a, b]$.

(ii) If $\sigma^2(x) = P(x) > 0$ is a polynomial in $[a, b]$ and $P^{(2m-1)}(x)$ has no zeroes in (a, b), then $q^{(2m-1)}(x) = (m - \gamma)P^{(2m-1)}(x)$ has no zeroes in $[a, b]$. Therefore, $\psi(x, \xi) - \gamma = q(x)\sigma^{-2}(x)$ has at most $2m - 1$ zeroes in $[a, b]$.

(iii) Then the degree of $q(x)$ is at most $2(m - 1)$ and therefore $\psi(x, \xi) - \gamma$ has at most $2m - 1$ zeroes in $[a, b]$.

(iv) Previous statements stay in the limit.

□

Later on, Wong (1993) proved this same result for minimax linear criteria of the type

$$\Phi(\xi) = \max_{z \in Z} \operatorname{tr}[B(z)M^{-1}(\xi)],$$

where Z is a compact set.

There are some interesting results relating Chebyshev systems and orthogonal polynomials with D-optimal designs. Theorem 3.5 states the D-optimal design ξ^* for the heteroscedastic polynomial regression models considered above has m points in its support, equally weighted. In some cases these points are the zeroe s of orthogonal polynomials $P_m(x)$ satisfying

$$\int_a^b P_i(x)P_j(x)\omega(x)dx = 0,\ i \neq j, \tag{3.6}$$

for some $\omega(x)$. For the typical classic orthogonal polynomials, (3.6) is satisfied if there exist polynomials $g_1(x)$ and $g_2(x)$ of degrees no larger than 1 and 2,

Table 3.1 Classic orthogonal polynomials with the respective characteristic functions

Family	$\omega(x)$	$g_2(x)$	$g_1(x)$	a_m	χ
Legendre	1	$1-x^2$	$-2x$	$m(m+1)$	$[-1,1]$
Hermite	e^{-x^2}	1	$-2x$	$2m$	$\mathbb{R}$
Laguerre	e^{-x}	x	$1-x$	m	$[0,\infty)$
General Laguerre	$x^\alpha e^{-x}$	x	$-(\alpha+1-x)$	$m-\alpha$	$[0,\infty)$
Chebyshev	$(1-x^2)^{-1/2}$	$1-x^2$	$-x$	m^2	$[-1,1]$
Jacobi	$(1-x)^\alpha(1+x)^\beta$	$1-x^2$	$\beta-\alpha-(\alpha+\beta+2)x$	$m(m+\alpha+\beta+1)$	$[-1,1]$

respectively, and a scalar a_m such that the *hypergeometric differential equation* is fulfilled,

$$g_2(x)P_m''(x)+g_1(x)P_m'(x)+a_mP_m(x)=0. \tag{3.7}$$

Table 3.1 shows some classic orthogonal polynomials with the form of $\omega(x)$, $g_1(x)$, $g_2(x)$, and a_m. Let $x_0,\ldots,x_{m-1}$ be the support points of the D-optimal design. If $P_{m-1}(x)=\prod_{i=0}^{m-1}(x-x_i)$ satisfies (3.7) for some functions $g_1(x)$ and $g_1(x)$ and some scalar a_m, then it will be some of the classic orthogonal polynomials. The D-optimal design maximizes

$$\det M(\xi^*)=\prod_{k=0}^{m-1}\xi^*(x_k)\prod_{r=0}^{m-1}\sigma^{-2}(x_r)\left|\prod_{i<j}^{m-1}(x_i-x_j)\right|.$$

This means the weights and the points are optimized independently and the weights are maximized for equal values. The logarithm is an increasing function so maximizing the determinant is equivalent to maximizing the log-determinant. Therefore, the derivative of the logarithm of the determinant with respect to the points has to be zero. Thus, we have these equations

$$\begin{aligned}0&=\frac{\lambda'(x_k)}{\lambda(x_k)}+\sum_{i\neq k}^{m-1}\frac{1}{x_k-x_i}\\&=\frac{\lambda'(x_k)\prod_{i\neq k}^{m-1}(x_k-x_i)+\lambda(x_k)\sum_{i\neq k}^{m-1}\prod_{l\neq i}^{m-1}(x_k-x_l)}{\lambda'(x_k)\prod_{i\neq k}^{m-1}(x_k-x_i)},\ k=0,\ldots,m-1,\end{aligned}$$

and therefore,

$$0=\lambda'(x_k)\prod_{i\neq k}^{m-1}(x_k-x_i)+\lambda(x_k)\sum_{i\neq k}^{m-1}\prod_{l\neq i}^{m-1}(x_k-x_l),\ k=0,\ldots,m-1. \tag{3.8}$$

These equations can be used to prove that Eq. (3.7) it satisfied at the m design points. These are the derivatives of $P_{m-1}(x)$,

$$P'_{m-1}(x) = \sum_r \prod_{i \neq r} (x - x_i), \qquad P'_{m-1}(x_k) = \prod_{i \neq k} (x_k - x_i),$$

$$P''_{m-1}(x) = \sum_r \sum_{i \neq r} \prod_{l \neq i,r} (x - x_l), \; P''_{m-1}(x_k) = \sum_{i \neq k} \prod_{l \neq i,k} (x_k - x_l).$$

The degree of $P_{m-1}(x)$ is $m - 1$. Then it is determined by m points. Thus, if Eq. (3.7) is satisfied for the m points, then $P_{m-1}(x)$ must satisfy the equation for all points.

Remark 3.5 These are some practical ideas around this:

1. The hypergeometric differential equation claims for $g_1(x)$ and $g_2(x)$ to be polynomials of degree 2 and 1, respectively, at most. Following the proof of the theorem it would be enough if $g_1(x) = g(x)p_1(x)$ and $g_1(x) = g(x)p_2(x)$ for some function $g(x)$, being $p_1(x)$ and $p_2(x)$ polynomials of degree 2 and 1, respectively. At the same time they should be of the form $g_1(x) = h(x)\lambda'(x)$, $g_2(x) = h(x)\lambda(x)$ for some $h(x)$ at the m design points.
2. This result allows the computation of some specific heteroscedastic polynomial models in specific design spaces.
3. Although usually the design space has to be assumed compact to guarantee the existence of an optimal design, a noncompact space "big enough" may still guarantee the existence of an optimal design.

Theorem 3.6 *Let a polynomial model satisfying*

(i) $\sigma^2(x) = 1,\ \chi = [-1, 1]$.
(ii) $\sigma^2(x) = (1 - x)^{\alpha-1}(1 + x)^{\beta-1},\ \chi = [-1, 1],\ \alpha, \beta < 1$.
(iii) $\sigma^2(x) = e^x,\ \chi = [0, \infty)$.
(iv) $\sigma^2(x) = x^{-(\alpha+1)}e^x,\ \chi = [0, \infty),\ \alpha > -1$.
(v) $\sigma^2(x) = e^{x^2},\ \chi = (-\infty, \infty)$.
(vi) $\sigma^2(x) = (1 - x^2)^{1/2-\alpha},\ \chi = [-1, 1],\ \alpha > -1/2$.

In all these cases there is a unique D-optimal design with m points in its support and they are zeros of the following orthogonal polynomials:

(i) $(1 - x^2)\frac{\partial P_{m-1}}{\partial x}$, *where* $P_{m-1}(x)$ *is the Legendre polynomial of degree* $m - 1$.
(ii) Jacobi polynomial $P^m_{\alpha,\beta}(x)$.
(iii) $xL^{(1)}_{m-1}(x)$, *where* $L^{(1)}_{m-1}(x)$ *is the Laguerre polynomial.*
(iv) $L^{(\alpha)}_m(x)$.
(v) Hermite polynomial $H_m(x)$.
(vi) Ultraspheric (Greenbauer) polynomial $C^{(\alpha)}_m(x)$.

Proof Table 3.1 shows the classic orthogonal polynomials with the respective characteristic functions. The proof of this Corollary is based on the well-known results summarized in this table. □

3.10 Correlated Observations and Spatiotemporal Models

All the theory of optimal experimental designs is quite elegant and clear for linear models. For nonlinear models the approximation of the covariance matrix of the estimators of the parameters by using the Fisher Information Matrix extends all the results with the important drawback that the FIM depends on the unknown parameters and something has to be done with that. The approximation is based on the Central Limit Theorem and then only applicable to uncorrelated observations. But a number of interesting problems account for some kind of correlation, for example, temporal or spatial. In Sect. 3.1 a general parametric model trying to describe a relationship between explanatory and response variables was established as a parametric family of distributions defined by the pdf

$$\{h(y_1, y_2, \dots, y_n \mid x_1, x_2, \dots, x_n; \theta_1, \theta_2, \dots, \theta_m) \mid \theta = (\theta_1, \theta_2, \dots, \theta_m)^T \in \Theta\}.$$

This definition includes the possible correlated observations case, but then the theory of approximate designs falls down as will be commented later. For a general model the parameters of the distribution family may be modeled through the explanatory variables and new parameters. For uncorrelated observations, typically the mean of the response, and the variance for the heteroscedastic case, can be modeled in this way. For correlated observations the covariance structure needs to be modeled as well. From a theoretical point of view, any mathematical expression can be used to model the mean. For the variance the mathematical expression has to be positive for all possible values of the explanatory variables. But, for the covariance just some particular mathematical functions can be used. They have to provide a positive definite covariance structure.

The typical time series models, such as autoregressive integrated moving average (ARIMA), are defined in a recurrent way relating the current observation with previous observations. In this case the covariance structure is implicit in the model and then this is not an issue from an estimation point of view, but it is from a design perspective. Amo-Salas et al. (2015) considered this type of models extracting explicitly the covariance structure from the model.

There is an extensive literature on design optimality for correlated observations under the so-called spatial statistics framework, for which the reader is referred to the book of Müller (2007b), while the paper by Müller and Stehlík (2009) offers interesting issues on this type of models and the corresponding optimal designs. Additionally, Pázman (2010) gave explicit expressions of the amount of information coming from a subset of the support of a given design. For correlated observations, the covariance structure is usually considered as temporally symmetric or spatially isotropic (i.e., spherically symmetric) function. In optimal design theory, crucial arguments are given by the Cramer–Rao theorem and the asymptotic approximation of the inverse of the Fisher Information Matrix to the covariance matrix of the MLEs of the parameters. Such arguments work well for uncorrelated observations, while for correlated the use of the FIM needs some justification. If the parameters of the mean are different from those of the covariance structure, there is still a justification for the use of the FIM for computing optimal designs (e.g., Pázman, 2004). The paper by Ying (1993) provides asymptotic properties of the estimates for computer experiments in a complete lattice-type design in the same situation. There is a version of the Central Limit Theorem for a type of weak correlation, which provides new insights for the justification of the FIM.

Actually, we do not need a good approximation of the covariance matrix by the inverse of the FIM. All we need for a particular criterion is a joint monotonicity between values of the criterion function for the covariance matrix and for the inverse of the FIM. For instance, consider D-optimality. Given two different designs, ξ_1 and ξ_2, then $\det M(\xi_1) \leq \det M(\xi_2)$ if and only if $\det \Sigma_{\hat{\theta}}(\xi_1) \geq \det \Sigma_{\hat{\theta}}(\xi_2)$. Last statement is not exact since $\Sigma_{\hat{\theta}}(\xi_i)$, $i = 1, 2$, depend on the observations. In that case we could assert the inequality for any possible sample of observations, the mean of the covariance matrix, or even the mean of the determinant, among other possibilities. Moreover, the FIM will depend on the parameters for a nonlinear model. This can be overcome by using the same estimates for each sample, some nominal values of the parameter or some prior distribution on the parameters.

All this could be no affordable from a theoretical point of view needing some numerical treatment. Thus, in a particular case (model, design space, and criterion), simulations can be performed on the different designs obtained along an algorithm for computing the optimal design. This can be done specially with the last designs obtained in the algorithm. Then the criterion function can be compered on the inverse of the FIMs and the covariance matrices to check whether both have similar decreasing behavior. Zhu and Stein (2005) performed some simulations to investigate the relationship between the inverse of the FIM and the covariance matrix of the MLE for the specific Matérn class of covariance structures when there is interest in estimating the parameters of both the mean and the covariance. Optimal designs for estimating mean and covariance are considered by Zhu and Zhang (2006) in a similar context. They stress that the asymptotic approximation of the inverse of the FIM and the covariance matrix of the MLEs are based on increasing domain asymptotic. Otherwise, the two matrices may behave differently.

Recently, Pázman et al. (2022) gave an interesting convex approach to optimum design of experiments with correlated observations allowing the use of approximate designs and providing a kind of equivalence theorem. This is very important for the computation of optimal designs.

3.10.1 Outline

Let $y(x_1), \ldots, y(x_n)$ a stochastic process defined as

$$y(x) = \eta(x; \theta) + \varepsilon(x), \qquad x \in \chi, \tag{3.9}$$

where θ is a vector of unknown parameters and $\varepsilon(\cdot)$ is usually a standard Gaussian process. This approach is justified, for example, by the literature on compartmental models, for which the reader is referred, for example, to Dette et al. (2006); Biedermann et al. (2007). In Amo-Salas et al. (2010), the authors assume a correlation of the exponential type between the observations. In general, a covariance structure has to be modeled. Typically, an *isotropic* structure is chosen $\mathrm{Cov}(y(x), y(z)) = C(h, \theta)$ with $h = ||x - z||$. This means the covariance depends on the explanatory variables, for example, time or space, through the distance between them. This natural isotropic property obliges the variance to be constant. Usually, C is decreasing on h, which is aligned with the fact that the correlation should decrease as one observation is farther from another.

Let $x_1, \ldots, x_n$ be an exact design, ξ, where some values may be repeated. The design can be considered as a discrete probability assigning weights to each point proportionally to the number of replications. Let X be the usual design matrix and let Σ_Y be the covariance matrix of the observations. If Σ_Y is known, then the FIM is

$$M(\xi, \theta) = X^T \Sigma_Y^{-1} X.$$

Even for this simple case the FIM is no longer additive. Therefore, neither Caratheodory's theorem nor the equivalence theorem satisfies anymore. Thus, a search for the optimal design has to be performed by using other type of algorithms, frequently with the convergence no guaranteed.

In a general case the FIM for all the parameters in the model, say θ, including parameters of the mean and the covariance matrix of the responses is

$$M(\xi, \theta) = \mathbf{E}_{\boldsymbol{\theta}} \left[\frac{\partial^2 \log h(y|x, \theta)}{\partial \theta^2} \right],$$

where $x = (x_1, \ldots, x_n)^T$, $y = (y(x_1), \ldots, y(x_n))^T$, $\eta(x, \theta) = (\eta(x_1, \theta), \ldots, \eta(x_n, \theta))^T$ and

$$\log h(y|x, \theta) = -\frac{1}{2} \Big[(y - \eta(x; \theta))^T \Sigma_Y^{-1}(\theta)(y - \eta(x; \theta)) + \log \det(\Sigma_Y(\theta)) + n \log(2\pi) \Big],$$

is the log-likelihood function of model (3.9). Arguments in Pázman (2004) show that

$$M(\xi, \theta) = \frac{\partial \eta^T(x;\theta)}{\partial \theta} \Sigma_Y^{-1}(\theta) \frac{\partial \eta(x;\theta)}{\partial \theta^T} + \frac{1}{2} \mathrm{tr} \left\{ \Sigma_Y^{-1}(\theta) \frac{\partial \Sigma_Y(\theta)}{\partial \theta} \Sigma_Y^{-1}(\theta) \frac{\partial \Sigma_Y(\theta)}{\partial \theta^T} \right\}, \tag{3.10}$$

where $\Sigma_Y(\theta)$ is the $n \times n$ matrix whose generic (i, j) entry is defined as $\Sigma_{ij}(\theta) = \mathrm{C}(x_i, x_j)$, with C being the covariance function and $\frac{\partial \Sigma_Y(\theta)}{\partial \theta}$ is a tensor (three-dimensional matrix $n \times m \times n$). Thus, the resulting product of the second summand can be seen as a $n \times n$ diagonal matrix with $m \times m$ matrices as elements. The symbol tr applies here as the sum of these diagonal matrices resulting a final $m \times m$ matrix.

3.10.2 Typical Models for the Covariance Structure

Amo-Salas et al. (2013) provided the theory to construct positive definite covariance structures in a practical way. In particular, the big family of Bernstein functions may generate a possible number for positive definite functions for selecting a proper covariance structure. I believe this is a very useful result to model correlation structures. In what follows some typical examples of isotropic covariance structures used in the literature are provided. In all of them h stands for the distance between the explanatory variables values where the experiments were realized. For instance, if the explanatory variable is time then

$$C(h; \theta) = \mathrm{Cov}(y(t), y(s)), \qquad \text{where } h = |t - s|.$$

Actually the h can be substituted by other quantities, such as the model mean under some conditions.

(i) Exponential (Cressie 1993)

$$C(h; \sigma^2, \delta) = \sigma^2 \exp\{-\delta h\}, \qquad h \geq 0, \tag{3.11}$$

where $\delta,\ \sigma^2 > 0$.

(ii) Triangular (Abt 1998)

$$C(h; \sigma^2, \rho) = \begin{matrix} \sigma^2(1 - h/\rho), & h \leq \rho, \\ 0, & h \geq \rho \end{matrix} \tag{3.12}$$

where $\rho,\ \sigma^2 > 0$.

(iii) Matérn function (Matérn 1986)

$$\varphi(h; \phi, \gamma) = (\phi h)^\gamma \mathcal{K}_\gamma(\phi h), \tag{3.13}$$

where γ, $\phi > 0$, and $\mathcal{K}_\gamma(\cdot)$ are the modified Bessel function of second kind. The Matérn model admits some special cases: $\varphi(h; \phi, 1/2) = \phi^{1/2}\sqrt{\frac{\pi}{2}}\exp(-\phi h)$ corresponds to the exponential model, that is, the covariance function associated to the Ornstein–Uhlenbeck process; $\varphi(h; \phi, \infty) = \exp(-\phi^2 h^2)$ is the so-called Gaussian model. The choice $\varphi(h; \phi, 3/2)$ corresponds to the covariance of an auto-regressive process of the third order.

(iv) Dagum function (Berg et al., 2008)

$$\varphi(h; \phi, \gamma) = 1 - \left(\frac{h^\phi}{1 + h^\phi}\right)^\gamma, \tag{3.14}$$

where $0 < \phi \leq 2$ and $0 < \gamma \leq 1$.

(v) Cauchy function (Gneiting and Schlather, 2004)

$$\varphi(h; \phi, \gamma) = (1 + h^\phi)^{-\gamma}, \tag{3.15}$$

where $0 < \phi \leq 2$ and $\gamma > 0$.

3.10.3 *Coordinate Descent Algorithm*

For exact designs the equivalence theorem is not satisfied (see, e.g., Atkinson et al., 2007a, §9.3). A commonly used algorithm for computing optimal exact designs is the so-called *coordinate descent* algorithm, very much used nowadays. It can also be applied to any objective function, usually for a multidimensional problem. The idea is as simple as fixing all the coordinates but one and optimize that one. Then repeat it with the rest of the coordinates, one by one. Thus, a one-dimensional optimization problem is solved at each step. Convergence is not guaranteed and there is a strong dependence on the initial values chosen to start the algorithm.

Brimkulov et al. (1986) provided an algorithm of this type by finding D-optimal sampling points by estimating parameters in linear models for expectations of random fields. A general scheme of the algorithm for D-optimality with correlated observations is detailed, in English, by Ucinski and Atkinson (2004). The algorithm starts from an arbitrary initial n-point design. In the case of exact optimal designs, the number of trials or points of the design is fixed by the practitioner and none of the points is repeated. At each iteration one support point is deleted from the current design and a new point is included in its place to maximize the value of the criterion function. The algorithm is detailed below step by step,

Step 1. Select an initial exact design $\xi_n^{(0)} = \{x_1^{(0)}, \ldots, x_n^{(0)}\}$ such that $x_i^{(0)} \neq x_j^{(0)}$ for $i \neq j \in I = \{1, 2, \ldots, n\}$.

Step 2. Given a design $\xi_n^{(s)}$ obtained at step s determine

$$(i^*, x^*) = \arg \min_{(i,x)\in I\times\chi} \Phi(\xi^{(s)}_{n,x_i\rightleftarrows x}),$$

where $\xi^{(s)}_{n,x_i\rightleftarrows x}$ means the support point x_i in design $\xi_n^{(s)}$ is changed by $x \in \chi$.

Step 3. Let $\xi_n^{(s+1)} = \xi^{(s)}_{n,x_{i^*}\rightleftarrows x^*}$.

Step 4. If $\frac{|\Phi(\xi_n^{(s)})-\Phi(\xi_n^{(s+1)})|}{\Phi(\xi_n^{(s)})} \leq \delta$, where δ is the given tolerance, then stop. Otherwise, set $s \leftarrow s+1$ and go to Step 2.

3.10.4 Examples

An exponential trend with exponential covariance is considered here,

$$y = \theta_1 e^{-\theta_2 t} + \varepsilon,$$

where the errors follow a normal distribution with mean zero and the covariance function depends just on the distance between the observations,

$$c(h) = \text{cov}(t, t+h) = \sigma^2 e^{-\theta_3 t}.$$

We consider a design space $\chi = [0, B]$ with B big enough to catch possible interior optimal points. For the uncorrelated case, the FIM at point t is

$$e^{-2\theta_2 t}\begin{pmatrix} 1 & \theta_1 t \\ \theta_1 t & \theta_1^2 t^2 \end{pmatrix}.$$

In this example we will always assume nominal values $\theta_1 = \theta_2 = 1$. The D-optimal design for the uncorrelated model is equally weighted at 0 and 1, no matter what the value of B would be. Figure 3.3 shows how the equivalence theorem is numerically satisfied.

For the correlated model two different scenarios are being considered.

σ^2 and θ_3 known: In this case the information matrix is $X^T\Sigma_Y^{-1}X$ with Σ_Y completely known and optimal designs do not depend on σ^2. For two points, say t and $t+h$,

$$\Sigma_Y = \sigma^2\begin{pmatrix} 1 & e^{-\theta_3 t} \\ e^{-\theta_3 t} & 1 \end{pmatrix}.$$

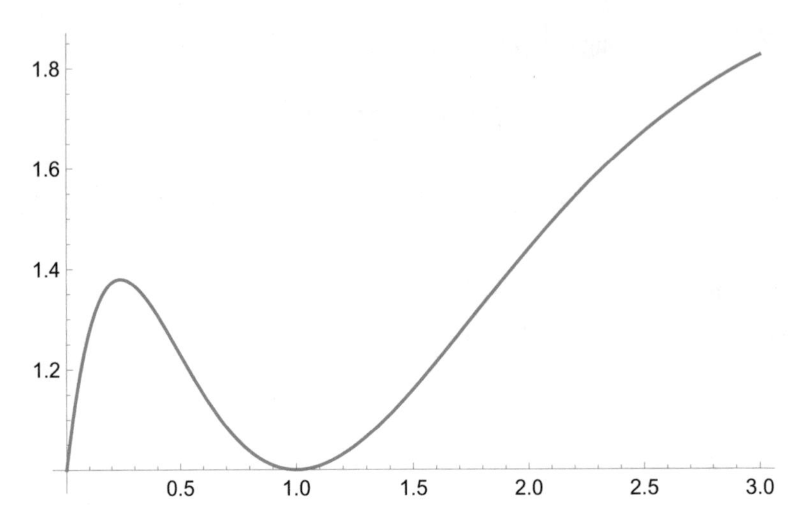

Fig. 3.3 Sensitivity function for the D-optimal design

Table 3.2 Two- and three-point exact D-optimal designs

θ_3	Two-point design	Three-point design
1	0, 0.797	0, 0.509, 1.306
10	0, 0.992	0, 0.741, 1.479

Table 3.3 Two-point exact D-optimal designs

θ_3	σ^2	Two-point design
1	0.5	0, 0.453
1	2	0, 0.404
3	0.5	0, 0.382
3	2	0, 0.365

Both for a two-point or a three-point exact D-optimal design point $t = 0$ is in it. Table 3.2 shows different results.

σ^2 and θ_3 unknown: This is the more realistic situation. Now the FIM is 4×4 since there are two extra columns and rows for the unknown parameters of the covariance structure. Now the optimal designs will depend on the variance σ^2 (Table 3.3).

There is not a way to check whether a particular exact design is or not optimal apart from direct computations or number theory.

3.11 Exercises

Exercise 3.1 Compute "universal" optimal designs for the model $y = e^{\theta x} + \varepsilon$, $x \in \chi = [a, b]$, $a > 0$, assuming a Gaussian distribution of the response with constant variance and nominal value $\theta_0 > 0$.

Solution $\begin{Bmatrix} b \\ 1 \end{Bmatrix}$.

Exercise 3.2 Let the model $y = \theta_1 x e^{-\theta_2 x^2} + \varepsilon$, $x \in \chi = [0, 1]$, assuming a Gaussian distribution of the response with constant variance. Previous experience provides information to use the nominal values $\theta_1 = 1$ y $\theta_2 = 5$.

1. Find the Fisher Information Matrix for the design

$$\xi_0 = \begin{Bmatrix} 0.5 & 1 \\ 1/5 & 4/5 \end{Bmatrix}.$$

Solution The FIM is

$$\begin{pmatrix} 0.00414057 & -0.00106238 \\ -0.00106238 & 0.000292836 \end{pmatrix}$$

2. Prove this is not a D-optimal design using the equivalence theorem and provide a bound for the D-efficiency.

Solution Figure 3.4 shows the sensitivity is not always positive. The bound for the efficiency is $2 - \frac{\max_{x\in[0,1]} f^T(x)M^{-1}(\xi)f(x)}{2} = -33.6897$, which is useless since the design is too far from being optimal.

3. Compute the D-optimal design assuming it is a two-point design.

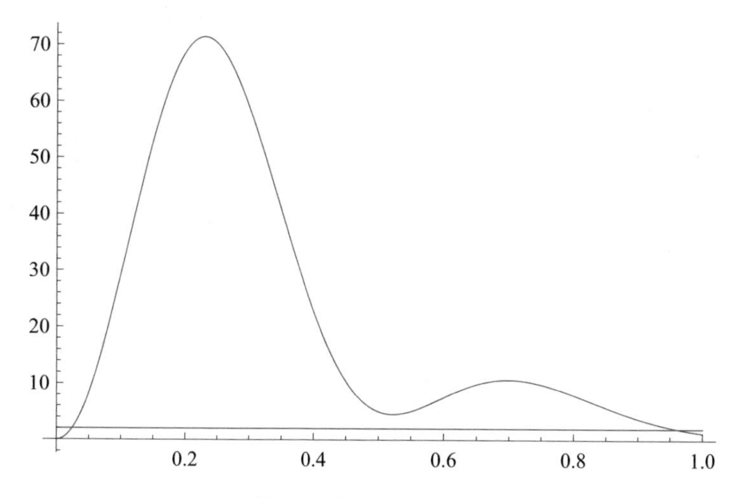

Fig. 3.4 Sensitivity function $2 - f^T(x)M^{-1}(\xi)f(x)$

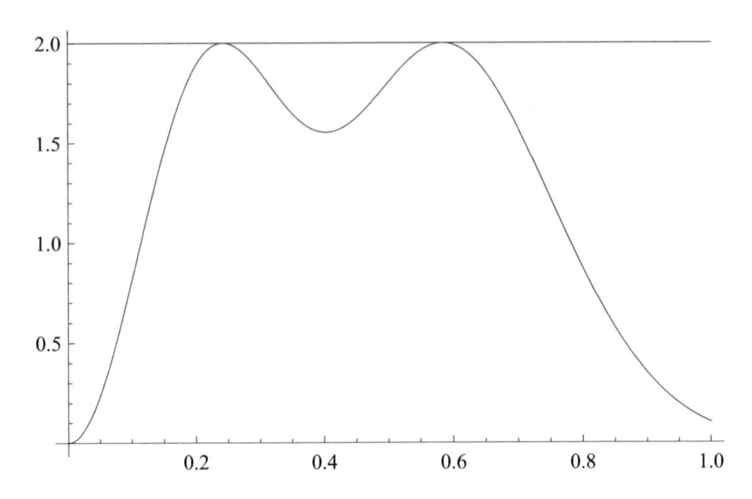

Fig. 3.5 Sensitivity function $f^T(x)M^{-1}(\xi)f(x)$

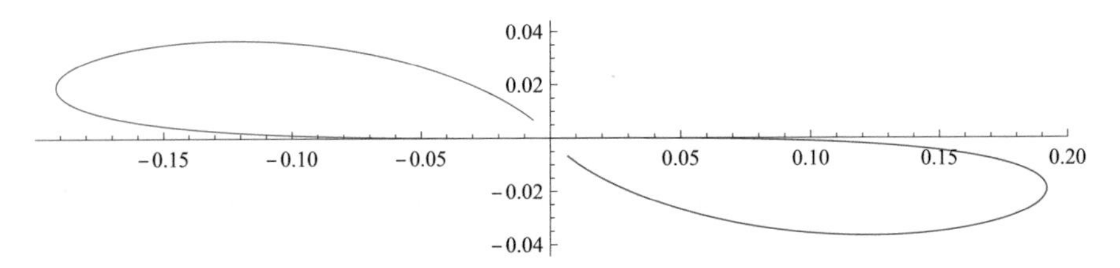

Fig. 3.6 Elfving set

Solution The two-point design maximizing the determinant of the FIM is

$$\left\{ \begin{matrix} \sqrt{\frac{1}{10}\left(2-\sqrt{2}\right)} = 0.24203 & \sqrt{\frac{1}{10}\left(2+\sqrt{2}\right)} = 0.584313 \\ 1/2 & 1/2 \end{matrix} \right\}.$$

For this design Fig. 3.5 shows $f^T(x)M^{-1}(\xi)f(x)$ is always under 2 reaching the zero just at the design points.

4. Compute c-optimal designs for $c = (1, 0)$ and (0, 1).

Solution Figure 3.6 shows the Elfving locus for computing c-optimal designs. Tangential points, t for the curve $f(t)$ and s for the curve $-f(s)$, are solutions of the equations:

$$\frac{x(t)+x(s)}{-x'(s)} = \frac{y(t)+y(s)}{-y'(s)}$$

$$\frac{x'(t)}{-x'(s)} = \frac{y'(t)}{-y'(s)}$$

giving the values $t^* = 0.222984$ and $s^* = 0.705541$, providing the support of the c-optimal design,

$$\begin{Bmatrix} 0.222984 & 0.705541 \\ 1 - p_c^* & p_c^* \end{Bmatrix}$$

For $c = (1, 0)$ the cut point is the root of the second component of the vector $(1 - p^*_{(1,0)}) f(t^*) - p^*_{(1,0)} f(s^*) = (A, 0)$, that is, $p^*_{(1,0)} = 0.228772$. For $c = (0, 1)$ it comes from the root of the first component of $(1 - p^*_{(0,1)}) f(t^*) - p^*_{(0,1)} f(s^*) = (0, B)$, that is, $p^*_{(0,1)} = 0.748093$.

Exercise 3.3 This is a classical model in pharmacokinetics,

$$y = \theta_1[1 - \exp(-\theta_2 x)] + \varepsilon,\ \varepsilon \sim \mathcal{N}(0, \sigma^2).$$

Compute D- and A-optimal designs.

Exercise 3.4 Let us consider logistic regression for one variable,

$$P(y = 1|x, \theta_1, \theta_2) = \frac{1}{1 + e^{-\theta_1 + \theta_2 x}}].$$

Compute D- and A-optimal designs assuming a big design space for nominal values of the parameters $\theta_1 = \theta_2 = 1$.

Solution Assuming a two-point design with equal weights and proving the equivalence theorem a D-optimal design are

$$\xi_D^\star = \begin{Bmatrix} -2.5434 & 0.5434 \\ 1/2 & 1/2 \end{Bmatrix}.$$

For A-optimality a two-point design with general weights can be assumed. Then the optimal weights can be computed using the formulae from Pukelsheim and Torsney (1991) (see Sect. 2.4.5 of this book) for two general points. Then the computed, and proving the equivalence theorem an A-optimal design is

$$\xi_D^\star = \begin{Bmatrix} -2.48231 & 0.482306 \\ 1/2 & 1/2 \end{Bmatrix},$$

which is not far from the D-optimal design.

Exercise 3.5 Let the model

$$y = \theta + \varepsilon,\ \varepsilon \sim \mathcal{N}(0, \sigma^2).$$

with correlated observations with covariance known structure

$$c(h) = \text{cov}(y(x), y(x+h)) = \sigma^2 e^{-h},$$

and design space $\chi = [a, b]$ with $a > 0$. Compute two- and three-point "universal" optimal exact designs assuming σ^2 is unknown and it has to be estimated.

Solution The log-likelihood for n points is

$$\ell(\theta) = -\frac{n}{2}\log(2\pi) - \frac{1}{2}\log(\det \Sigma_n) - \frac{1}{2}(Y - \Theta)^T \sigma^{-1}(Y - \Theta),$$

where $Y^T = (y_1, \ldots, y_n)$ and $\Theta^T = (\theta, \ldots, \theta)$.

The covariance matrices for two and three points, say $x, x+h$ (and $x+h+r$), are

$$\Sigma_Y = \sigma^2 \begin{pmatrix} 1 & e^{-h} \\ e^{-h} & 1 \end{pmatrix}, \qquad \Sigma_Y = \sigma^2 \begin{pmatrix} 1 & e^{-h} & e^{-h-r} \\ e^{-h} & 1 & e^{-r} \\ e^{-h-r} & e^{-r} & 1 \end{pmatrix}.$$

After deriving ℓ twice with respect to θ and σ^2 and computing the expectation of the opposite of the FIMs are, respectively,

$$\sigma^{-2} \begin{pmatrix} \frac{2e^h}{1+e^h} & 0 \\ 0 & 1 \end{pmatrix}, \qquad \sigma^{-2} \begin{pmatrix} 3 - \frac{2}{1+e^h} - \frac{2}{1+e^r} & 0 \\ 0 & 3/2 \end{pmatrix}.$$

The optimal design does not depend on σ^2 and one point is enough for estimating both parameters. For two points the first component increases with the distance of the two points, h; thus, the optimal design is $\xi = \{a, b\}$. For three points the optimal design is $\xi = \{a, \frac{a+b}{2}, b\}$.

Chapter 4
Bayesian Optimal Designs

4.1 Introduction

Chaloner and Verdinelli (1995) reviewed this topic in a long and rigorous work both for linear and nonlinear models. Under the Bayesian paradigm of the decision theory, many optimality criteria are justified and new approaches are opened. DasGupta (2007) presented a complementary review of Bayesian optimal design. A typical criticism to the design of experiments is that some assumptions such as the model or the optimality criterion have to be made before collecting the data. Another criticism for nonlinear models is that the Fisher Information Matrix depends on the unknown parameters to be estimated. Some of the solutions proposed in the literature for this inconvenience include the use of locally optimal designs for some nominal values of the parameters, sequential designs improving the estimators of the parameters during the process, or Bayesian designs for some prior distribution of the parameters. Bayesian design of experiments seeks for taking advantage of the information that is available prior to experimentation, to design optimally the experiments to be realized. A rigorous approach from a decision theory point of view may help with all this.

Brooks (1972, 1976) motivated the problem of choosing the best subset of regressors and the design points in a linear regression model. Here predicting the future value of the dependent variable was the goal of the experiment and the predictor was obtained substituting the Bayesian estimator in the regression function rather than considering the prediction distribution for the future observation. Bayesian optimality criteria have frequently been considered as particular linear criteria (e.g., Fedorov 1972; Pukelsheim 1993; Pilz 1993). In particular, Pilz (1993) showed Bayesian criteria as limiting cases when diffuse prior information is considered.

Pilz (1993) offered a very general approach with no distributional assumptions for the model or for the prior. In that book, the Bayesian alphabetical optimality criteria were defined as an extension of the corresponding non-Bayesian criteria and looked at them as special cases of a general linear optimality criteria. D-optimality

J. López-Fidalgo, *Optimal Experimental Design*, Lecture Notes in Statistics 226,
https://doi.org/10.1007/978-3-031-35918-7_4

and E-optimality do not fall into this setting and they are derived separately. Pilz (1993) used the classical decision theory considering admissible and complete classes of designs to find conditions for the existence of Bayesian designs in an admissible class. He also uses Whittle's general version of the equivalence theorem (Whittle, 1973) to find relationships between the different design criteria and to construct bounds for the designs. He shows that under certain conditions Bayesian alphabetical criteria can be seen as L-optimal designs for a transformed model.

Let $\pi(\theta)$ be a prior distribution of the vector of unknown parameters, θ. In what follows just π and h will be used for either marginal, conditional, or joint distributions on θ and observations, respectively. Using the approach given by Lindley and Smith (1972) (pp 19–20), the problem is reduced to finding the design that maximizes the expected utility of the experiment outcome. The optimal design problem is then determined by the expected utility of the best decision,

$$\xi^\star = \arg\max_{\xi\in\Xi} U(\xi) = \arg\max_{\xi\in\Xi} \int_{\mathcal{Y}} \max_{d\in\mathcal{D}} \int_{\Theta} U(d,\theta,\xi,y)\pi(\theta|y,\xi)h(y|\xi)d\theta dy,$$

where Θ is the parameters space, $U(d,\theta,\xi,y)$ is the utility function chosen to satisfy certain goal, y is the vector of the responses from a sample space $\mathcal{Y}$, $h(y|\xi)$ is a suitable marginal density for the response, $\pi(\theta|y,\xi)$ is the posterior pdf, and d is a decision on the model, typically the estimators of the parameters. Since

$$\pi(\theta|y,\xi) = \frac{\pi(\theta|y,\xi)h(y|\theta\xi)}{h(y|\xi)},$$

the annoying marginal distribution $h(y|\xi)$ does not depend on θ and disappears in many practical computations.

Notice that the data are the observations y jointly with the associated design ξ. Thus, the decision is being made in two steps: first, selection of ξ and then the choice of an optimal estimator of the parameters, d. Since at the time of selecting the design the observations y are unknown, the expected utility function has to be considered not only on the parameters but also on the observations. Once the experiment is performed and the data is known we go back to the utility function without the need of the expectation on the distribution of the observations.

There are two important things to be assumed in this problem. On the one hand, a prior distribution of the parameters has to be given. On the other hand, a utility joint function has to be specified both for appropriately describing the goals of a given experiment and for estimating the parameters. The choice of a utility or loss function expresses various reasons for carrying out an experiment. In the linear model the widely known non-Bayesian alphabetical design criteria have some theoretical justification. In the Bayesian framework, when inference about the parameters is the main goal of the analysis, a utility function based on Shannon information leads to Bayesian D-optimality in the normal linear model (Bernardo, 1979). In addition, Shannon information can be used for prediction and also mixing utility functions for describing several simultaneous goals for an experiment. Some but not all the alphabetical optimality criteria have a utility-based Bayesian version. Several utility functions and prior distributions will be considered in the next sections.

4.2 Linear Models

A linear model, that is, Independent Normal observations with constant variance and a mean linear on the parameters, will be considered in what follows with the typical approach given in Sect. 2.1. Let X be the $n \times m$ design matrix and let X_i^T, $i = 1, \ldots, n$ be the rows of X. The matrix $X^T X$ is often referred to as the information matrix. If n_i observations are taken at the point x_i, then the information matrix can be written as $n \sum_i \frac{n_i}{n} X_i X_i^T$, with $\sum_i \frac{n_i}{n} = 1$. Thus, if ξ is the corresponding measure of this particular exact design, then $nM(\xi) = X^T X$.

Both exact and approximate optimal designs will be considered depending on specific situations. In some cases, using a linear model, exact calculations for expected utility $U(d, \theta, \xi, y)$ are possible. For nonlinear models expected utilities do not have a closed-form representation and approximations are required.

Consider the problem of choosing an approximate design ξ. Let y be a vector of n observations where $y|\theta, \sigma^2 \sim \mathcal{N}(X\theta, \sigma^2 I)$, where θ is a vector of m unknown parameters, σ^2 is known, and I is the $n \times n$ identity matrix. Suppose that the prior information is such that $\theta|\sigma^2$ is normally distributed with mean $\theta^{(0)}$ and covariance matrix $\sigma^2 R^{-1}$ where the $m \times m$ matrix R is known. It is well-known that the posterior distribution for $\theta|\sigma^2$, that is, σ^2 is assumed known, is also normal with mean vector

$$\theta^\star = (X^T X + R)^{-1}(X^T y + R\theta^{(0)}) \tag{4.1}$$

and covariance matrix $\sigma^2(X^T X + R)^{-1}$. From now on $M_B(\xi) = M(\xi) + \frac{1}{n} R$ will be the so-called Bayesian Information Matrix.

Remark 4.1

1. If σ^2 is assumed unknown in a more realistic scenario, the outline is more complex. It will be considered later assuming a prior distribution also for σ^2.
2. If R is nonsingular then for a proper informative prior distribution $X^T X + R$ is nonsingular, even if rank$X < m$ and then $X^T X$ is singular. This means the optimal design could have less than m different points in its support.
   A proper informative distribution means a well-defined probability distribution. In Bayesian statistics, sometimes an improper noninformative prior distribution such as a uniform distribution in the whole real line with a constant "pseudo" pdf. Then using the Bayesian theorem the posterior distribution is standardized to be a proper one.

3. Using Caratheodory's theorem in the usual way, for any design ξ there is always a design ξ' such that $\#S_{\xi'} \leq m(m+1)/2 + 1$ and $M_B(\xi') = M_B(\xi)$. Here # stands for the cardinal, that is, the number of elements, of a set.
4. The set of Bayesian Information Matrices is convex.

4.2.1 *Criteria Derived from Particular Utility Functions*

One possible utility criterion is the expected Kullback–Leibler distance between the posterior and the prior distributions,

$$\begin{aligned}
&\mathrm{E}_y \left[\int \pi(\theta|y,\xi) \log \frac{\pi(\theta|y,\xi)}{\pi(\theta)} d\theta \right] \\
&= \int \int h(y|\xi) \frac{h(y,\theta|\xi)}{h(y|\xi) \times \log \frac{\pi(\theta|y,\xi)}{\pi(\theta)} d\theta dy} \\
&= \int \int h(y,\theta|\xi) \log \frac{\pi(\theta|y,\xi)}{\pi(\theta)} d\theta dy \\
&= \int \int h(y,\theta|\xi) \log \pi(\theta|y,\xi) d\theta dy - \int \int h(y,\theta|\xi) \log \pi(\theta) d\theta dy.
\end{aligned}$$

Lindley (1956), Stone (1959a, 1959b), DeGroot (1962, 1986), and Bernardo (1979) suggested considering the expected gain in Shannon information given by an experiment as a utility function (Shannon, 1948),

$$\int h(y,\theta|\xi) \log \pi(\theta|y,\xi) d\theta dy, \tag{4.2}$$

This is actually the first part of the Kullback–Leibler distance. This criterion focuses on the estimation of the parameters. In particular, for the normal linear regression model,

$$\begin{aligned}
\pi(\theta|y,\xi) = &\frac{1}{\sqrt{(2\pi)^m \det[\sigma^2 (X^T X + R)^{-1}]}} \\
&\times \exp\left[-\frac{1}{2} \frac{(\theta - \theta^\star)^T (X^T X + R)(\theta - \theta^\star)}{\sigma^2} \right],
\end{aligned}$$

and the expression (4.2) becomes

$$\mathrm{E}_h\mathrm{E}_{\pi(\cdot|y,\xi)}\left\{-\frac{1}{2}\left[m\log 2\pi + \log\det\sigma^2(X^TX+R)^{-1}\right]\right.$$
$$\left.-\frac{1}{2}\frac{(\theta-\theta^\star)^T(X^TX+R)(\theta-\theta^\star)}{\sigma^2}\right\}$$
$$= -\frac{m}{2}\log(2\pi) - \frac{m}{2} + \frac{1}{2}\log\det\sigma^{-2}(nM(\xi)+R),$$

where it has been taken into account that for multivariate random vector u with mean μ_u and covariance matrix Σ_u

$$\begin{aligned}\mathrm{E}[(u-\mu_u)^T\Sigma_u^{-1}(u-\mu_u)] &= \mathrm{E}[\mathrm{tr}\Sigma_u^{-1}(u-\mu_u)(u-\mu_u)^T] \\ &= \mathrm{tr}\left\{\Sigma_u^{-1}\mathrm{E}[(u-\mu_u)(u-\mu_u)^T]\right\} \\ &= \mathrm{tr}[\Sigma_u^{-1}\Sigma_u] = m.\end{aligned}$$

Then, the optimality criterion reduces to minimizing

$$\Phi_D^B(\xi) = -\log\det\left[M(\xi) + \frac{1}{n}R\right].$$

This criterion may be considered as *Bayesian D-optimality*. There are other utility functions justifying this criterion. In particular, Spezzaferri (1988) obtained the same criterion from other utility function for model discrimination and parameter estimation. Other justification was given by Eaton et al. (1994) through utility functions based on proper scoring rules for prediction, where D-optimality is a special case. Finally, this Bayesian D-optimality criterion was derived by Tiao and Afonja (1976) from a two-valued utility function. Details are not provided here, but this reflects the justification of this criterion from different points of view.

If the interest is in estimating the parameters or linear combinations of them, a quadratic loss function might be appropriate,

$$-\int(\theta-\hat{\theta})^T HH^T(\theta-\hat{\theta})\pi(\theta|y,\xi)h(y|\theta,\xi)d\theta dy$$
$$= -\sigma^2\mathrm{tr}H^T\left[nM(\xi)+R\right]^{-1}H, \tag{4.3}$$

where H is a full rank $m \times l$ matrix. Using again (4.3) the Bayesian criterion can be defined as

$$\Phi_L^B(\xi) = \mathrm{tr}H^T\left[M(\xi) + \frac{1}{n}R\right]^{-1}H,$$

adapting L-optimality. Special cases are Bayesian A-optimality for $H = I$, the identity matrix,

$$\Phi_A^B(\xi) = \operatorname{tr}\left[M(\xi) + \frac{1}{n}R\right]^{-1},$$

and Bayesian c-optimality for a vector $H = c$,

$$\Phi_c^B(\xi) = c^T\left[M(\xi) + \frac{1}{n}R\right]^{-1} c.$$

If matrix HH^T is singular, as it happens in the previous case, the optimal design in the classic theory can be singular with a singular information matrix. Then the use of pseudo-inverses is needed. This is avoided for the Bayesian approach (Remark 4.1). If $\operatorname{rank}(W) = l$, then there is always a Bayesian L-optimal design with no more than $\frac{l(2m-l+1)}{2}$ points in its support.

For c-optimality a Bayesian modification of the geometric argument in Elfving's theorem (Elfving, 1952) was given by Chaloner (1984). Extended versions were provided by El Krunz and Studden (1991) and Dette (1993a, 1993b).

Bayesian E-optimality looks for the design minimizing the maximum posterior variance of all possible normalized linear combinations of parameter estimators. This is equivalent to minimizing the maximum eigenvalue of the posterior covariance matrix,

$$\Phi_E^B(\xi) = \sup_{||c||=1} c^T\left[M(\xi) + \frac{1}{n}R\right]^{-1} c = \lambda_{max}\left[M(\xi) + \frac{1}{n}R\right],$$

where λ_{max} stands for the maximum eigenvalue of the matrix. This criterion appears not to correspond to any utility function, and so although it is referred to as Bayesian E-optimality, its Bayesian justification in a decision theoretic context is unclear. Closely related to Bayesian E-optimality is Bayesian G-optimality,

$$\Phi_G^B(\xi) = \sup_{x\in\chi} f^T(x)\left[M(\xi) + \frac{1}{n}R\right]^{-1} f(x).$$

Similarly to E-optimality this does not correspond to maximizing a utility function although there is an equivalence theorem that states that approximate G-optimal designs are numerically identical to a corresponding approximate D-optimal design (Pukelsheim, 1993, §11.6). Tiao and Afonja (1976) considered other utility functions aimed at the problems of selecting the best of some parameters as well as ranking the parameters. They also proposed other utilities and considered the problem of choosing among a class of balanced designs to illustrate the use of the utilities and to show that a design often has to be selected from a limited range of available ones.

Remark 4.2 Since $M_B(\xi) = M(\xi) + \frac{1}{n}R$ depends on n, an optimal Bayesian design depends also on the sample size n. Moreover, any differences between a Bayesian design and its corresponding non-Bayesian one are unimportant if n is large. This is intuitively reasonable since in experiments where the sample size is large the posterior distribution will be driven by the data and will not be sensitive to the prior distribution. In contrast, if n is small the prior distribution could affect very much the posterior distribution. When there is little prior information available, optimal Bayesian designs are close to the corresponding non-Bayesian ones. Hence, when a noninformative prior distribution is used for inference as may often be the case, there is no advantage to using the Bayesian approach for design. This limiting behavior is not seen in design for nonlinear models where usual non-Bayesian optimal designs are again special cases of Bayesian design but correspond to a point mass prior distribution rather than noninformativeness. This is because here the FIM depends on the parameters.

When prediction is more important than estimation, the Bayesian approach needs a predictive analysis. For example, the expected gain in Shannon information on a future observation (prediction at x_{n+1}), say $\hat{y}_{n+1}$, can be used instead of the expected gain in information of the parameters. Let $h(\hat{y}_{n+1})$ be the prior distribution of the prediction. Then the Kullback–Leibler distance between the prior and the posterior prediction distribution is

$$\int h(\hat{y}_{n+1}|y,\xi) \log \frac{h(\hat{y}_{n+1}|y,\xi)}{h(\hat{y}_{n+1})} dy d\hat{y}_{n+1}.$$

Another possible utility function is the expected gain in Shannon information.

$$U(\xi) = \int h(\hat{y}_{n+1}|y,\xi) \log h(\hat{y}_{n+1}|y,\xi) dy d\hat{y}_{n+1}.$$

This utility function has been used by San Martini and Spezzaferri (1984) for a model selection problem and by Verdinelli et al. (1993) for accelerated life test experiments. In the normal linear model, this optimization problems correspond to maximizing

$$\begin{aligned} U(\xi) &= \mathrm{E}_{(y,\hat{y}_{n+1})}\left[\log h(\hat{y}_{n+1}|y,\xi)\right] \\ &= \mathrm{E}_{(y,\hat{y}_{n+1})}\left\{ \log\left[\frac{1}{\sqrt{2\pi\sigma^2\left[\frac{1}{n}x_{n+1}^T M_B^{-1}(\xi) x_{n+1} + 1\right]}} \right.\right. \end{aligned}$$

$$\left.\left.\times \exp\left\{\frac{(\hat{y}_{n+1}-\hat{x}_{n+1}^T\theta)^2}{2\sigma^2\left[\frac{1}{n}x_{n+1}^T M_B^{-1}(\xi)x_{n+1}+1\right]}\right\}\right]\right\}$$

$$= -\frac{1}{2}\left\{\log(2\pi)+1-\log\left[\frac{1}{n}\sigma^2 x_{n+1}^T M_B^{-1}(\xi)x_{n+1}+\sigma^2\right]\right\},$$

This is equivalent to minimizing the posterior prediction variance $x_{n+1}^T M_B^{-1}(\xi)x_{n+1}$. If the interest is in predicting just at a particular value, then the criterion is Bayesian c-optimality.

4.2.2 Unknown Variance

If σ^2 is assumed unknown in the linear model, then the optimality criteria induced by the utility functions of the earlier sections may need to be modified although conceptually the goal of maximizing a utility remains the same. If a gamma distribution is considered as the marginal prior of σ^2 with parameters α and β and the conditional prior of θ given σ^2 is a multivariate normal distribution with mean $\theta^{(0)}$ and covariance matrix $\sigma^2 R^{-1}$, then the posterior marginal distribution of σ^2 is again a Gamma distribution with parameters $\alpha^\star = \alpha + n/2$ and $\beta^\star = \beta + \frac{1}{2}[(Y - X\theta^\star)^T Y + (\theta^{(0)} - \theta^\star)^T R\theta^{(0)}]$, where θ^* is the mean of the posterior conditional distribution of θ given σ^2 in Eq. (4.1). Thus, the variance of the posterior marginal distribution is

$$\sigma_\star^2 = \frac{\alpha + n/2 + \beta^\star}{\alpha + n/2}.$$

The marginal prior and posterior distribution of θ are multivariate t distributions. Considering the covariance matrix of the vector of parameters including the variance makes the problem much more complex from an algebraic point of view. Brooks (1972) examined this case and used the simple solution to the problem that substitutes the value of σ^2 with its prior mean wherever it appears in the final expression of the criterion. This approach was also used by other authors such as Pukelsheim (1993) in chapter 11.

Denote by $t_\delta(m, \theta^{(0)}, R^{-1})$ the probability distribution of a multivariate random variable of dimension m with a t distribution with δ degrees of freedom, mean vector $\theta^{(0)}$, and scale matrix R^{-1}. Let $g(\xi, Y) = (2\alpha + n)^{-1}\left\{(Y - X\theta^{(0)})^T[I - X(nM(\xi)+R)^{-1}X^T](Y - X\theta^{(0)}) + 2\beta\right\}$ and let $a = \alpha/\beta$. The marginal prior and posterior distributions of θ are

$$\theta \sim t_{2\alpha}(m, \theta^{(0)}, aR^{-1}), \quad \theta \mid Y, \xi \sim t_{2\alpha+n}(m, \theta^*, g(\xi, Y)(nM(\xi)+R)^{-1}).$$

The distribution of Y conditional on θ is $t_{2\alpha}(n, X\theta, aI)$ and

$$Y|\xi \sim t_{2\alpha}\left\{n, X\theta^{(0)}, a[I - X(nM(\xi) + R)^{-1}X^T]^{-1}\right\}.$$

The posterior prediction distribution for a new observation $\hat{y}_{n+1}$ at x_{n+1} is then

$$\hat{y}_{n+1}|Y, \xi \sim t_{2\alpha+n}\left\{1, x_{n+1}\theta^*, g(\xi, Y)[x_{n+1}^T(nM(\xi) + R)^{-1}x_{n+1}] + 1\right\},$$

Evaluating the expected utilities presented in previous sections is now an intractable task since no closed-form expression can be derived. Numerical approaches or approximations such as normal approximations are needed. Things are somewhat simpler for A-optimality, where the derived criterion from the corresponding quadratic loss function (4.3) for $W = I$ reduces to $\int \Sigma_{\theta|Y}\pi(Y)dY$ maximizing the expression

$$\frac{-\alpha + n}{2\alpha + n - 2}\mathrm{tr}(nM(\xi) + R)^{-1}\int g(\xi, Y)\pi(y)dy,$$

where $\int g(\xi, Y)\pi(Y)dY = [2\beta n(2\alpha - 1)^{-1} + 2\beta]/(2\alpha + n)$, which does not depend on σ^2. Thus, Bayesian A-optimality is insensitive to the knowledge of σ^2.

4.3 Nonlinear Models

The model is said nonlinear either when the mean is modeled by a nonlinear function of the parameters or any of the conditions of normality, independence, or homoscedasticity fail. In this section we will consider the former case where some nonlinear function of the parameters needs to be estimated and the usual assumptions of normality, independence, or homoscedasticity are satisfied. Approximations must typically be used since a closed form of the exact expected utility is often impossible to obtain. Approximate or exact designs are still valid here. Most approximations to expected utility involve using a normal approximation to the posterior distribution, where the matrix of second derivatives of the logarithm of either the likelihood (FIM) or the posterior density appears.

Let $M(\xi, \theta)$ be the FIM, which it now depends on the parameters. Let $\hat{\theta}$ be the MLE of θ. Berger (1985) provided some normal approximations of the posterior distribution, for instance,

$$\theta|y, \xi \sim \mathcal{N}\left(\hat{\theta}, M^{-1}(\xi, \hat{\theta})\frac{\hat{\sigma}^2}{n}\right). \tag{4.4}$$

Another approximation is

$$\theta|y, \xi \sim \mathcal{N}\left(\hat{\theta}, [nM(\xi, \hat{\theta}) + R]^{-1}\hat{\sigma}^2\right), \tag{4.5}$$

where now $\hat{\theta}$ is the mode of the joint posterior distribution of θ, called the generalized maximum likelihood estimator of θ, and R is the matrix of second derivatives of the logarithm of the prior density function, which it is called the precision matrix of the prior distribution.

Several other approximations are possible, for example, using the exact posterior mean and variance as the mean and variance of the approximating normal distribution or using the observed rather than expected FIM. Although in specific problems there may be reasons to prefer one approximation to another, the observed FIM, rather than the expected, almost always gives a better normal approximation to the posterior distribution. In general, there is no obviously best one to use. For design purposes the expected FIM is usually algebraically much more tractable.

4.3.1 Shannon Information and Bayesian D-optimality

For the Shannon information the expected utility is given by the same equation as in the linear model involving the marginal distribution of the data for a design. In most cases this marginal distribution of y must also be approximated. When the posterior utility only depends on y through some consistent estimator $\hat{\theta}$, a further approximation of the same order as (4.4) and (4.5) is to take the prediction distribution of $\hat{\theta}$ to be the prior distribution. Using this approximation together with (4.4) gives an approximate value of the utility function,

$$-\frac{m}{2}\log 2\pi - \frac{m}{2} + \frac{1}{2}\int \log\det nM^{-1}(\xi, \theta)\pi(\theta)d\theta.$$

This gives the criterion

$$\Phi_D^{sB}(\xi) = \int \log\det M^{-1}(\xi, \theta)\pi(\theta)d\theta = E_\theta[\log\det M^{-1}(\xi, \theta)],$$

which does not depend on n and approximate designs can be used without the need of fixing the sample size.

Using (4.5) the criterion becomes

$$\Phi_D^B(\xi) = \int \log\det[nM(\xi, \theta) + R]^{-1}\pi(\theta)d\theta.$$

4.3.2 Bayesian c-Optimality

If we are interested in estimating a function g of the parameters and the squared error loss is appropriate, then vector

$$c(\theta) = \frac{\partial g(\theta)}{\partial \theta}$$

approximates locally the direction of the quantity to be estimated. Using (4.4), the utility function is

$$\Phi_c^{sB}(\xi) = \int c^T(\theta)M^{-1}(\xi,\theta)c(\theta)\pi(\theta)d\theta = E_\theta[c^T(\theta)M^{-1}(\xi,\theta)c(\theta)],$$

and using (4.5),

$$\Phi_c^{B}(\xi) = \int c^T(\theta)[nM(\xi,\theta)+R]^{-1}c(\theta)\pi(\theta)d\theta = E_\theta[c^T(\theta)M^{-1}(\xi,\theta)c(\theta)].$$

4.3.3 Bayesian L-optimality

If the interest is in estimating several functions, the total expected loss is the sum of the expected losses. This sum could be a weighted sum to represent some functions being of more interest than others. Let $W(\theta)$ be the matrix with the sum of the individual matrices of type $c(\theta)c^T(\theta)$, then the two typical approximate utilities as in previous sections are

$$\Phi_L^{sB}(\xi) = \int \mathrm{tr}[W(\theta)M^{-1}(\xi,\theta)]\pi(\theta)d\theta = E_\theta\{\mathrm{tr}[W(\theta)M^{-1}(\xi,\theta)]\},$$

and

$$\Phi_L^{B}(\xi) = \int \mathrm{tr}\left\{W(\theta)\right\}\pi(\theta)d\theta = E_\theta\left\{\mathrm{tr}[W(\theta)[nM(\xi,\theta)+R]^{-1}]\right\}.$$

4.3.4 Extended Bayesian Criteria

Following previous ideas two possible criteria may be considered for any non-Bayesian optimality criterion Φ to be minimized. On the one hand, let

$$\Phi^{sB}(\xi) = \mathrm{E}_\pi\left\{\Phi[M(\xi,\theta)]\right\}. \tag{4.6}$$

It is quite frequent to call it *pseudo-Bayesian optimality* criterion. Here the prior covariance matrix is not explicit in the integrated function. The second criterion involving this matrix is

$$\Phi^B(\xi) = \mathrm{E}_\pi \left\{ \Phi \left[M(\xi,\theta) + \frac{1}{n} R \right] \right\}. \tag{4.7}$$

For liner models the matrix does not depend on the parameters, so (4.6) is nothing else than the non-Bayesian criterion. Since the criterion function may have different forms, as is the case for D-optimality, different criteria may be considered if the expectation is taken with or without the log,

$$\Phi_D^{sB}(\xi) = -\mathrm{E}_\pi \left[\log \det M(\xi) \right], \tag{4.8}$$

$$\Phi_D^{sB}(\xi) = \mathrm{E}_\pi \left[\det M^{-1}(\xi) \right]. \tag{4.9}$$

The justification based on the Shanon information leads to the expectation of the log of the determinant, but taking into account that the determinant is proportional to the volume of the confidence ellipsoid, it may also make sense to use directly the expected value of the determinant.

Other two criteria can be generated adding the R. But there are still another two possibilities for any non-Bayesian criterion exchanging the FIM with its expectation or even more adequately exchanging the inverse of the FIM with its expectation. Both ways are very natural from a first sight of the problem, but they are rarely used since after the expectation of each entry of either the FIM or it inverse, the matrix may lose important properties. We will not use these definitions in this book.

Remark 4.3

1. For linear models Φ^{sB} is just the ordinary criterion.
2. All these criteria are nonincreasing in the Loewner sense. Since all these criteria are based on normal approximations, one may think in searching for designs to optimize also the approximations.
3. Since $M_B(\xi) = M(\xi) + \frac{1}{n} R$ depends on n, an optimal Bayesian design depends also on the sample size n.
4. If the prior is a one-point distribution, the Bayesian problem corresponds to locally optimal designs.
5. There are unimportant differences between Bayesian and non-Bayesian results if n is large.
6. If n is small the prior could affect very much the posterior.
7. If there is little prior information, then both are close.
8. This limiting behavior is not seen for nonlinear models (the FIM depends on the parameters).

9. Bayesian criteria for discriminating between models have been rarely considered in the literature. For instance, Spezzaferri (1988) used the utility function

$$U(\theta, \pi) = 2\pi(\theta) - \int \pi^2(\tau) d\tau, \tag{4.10}$$

for the dual goal of discriminating between two linear models and parameter estimation. For the dual purpose of model discrimination and parameter estimation for two nested normal linear models, the optimality criterion derived using (4.10) is given by the product of two factors. One is the determinant of the information matrix of the smaller model. The other factor is the expectation of the posterior probability of the smaller model when it is assumed to be true. Just for discriminating he derived a criterion minimizing the expectation of the posterior probability of one model, when the other was assumed true. Tommasi and López-Fidalgo (2010) used a Bayesian approach for discriminating between two models assuming a compound criterion for the two possible Kullback–Leibler distances.

4.4 Equivalence Theorem

In Sects. 2.6 and 2.6.1 the equivalence theorem was presented as an important and useful tool in OED. The question is whether this result can be used under the Bayesian paradigm and if so to what extent. Criteria (4.7) and (4.6) are convex if Φ is convex, both for linear and nonlinear models. Then the equivalence theorem can be extended straightforward for Bayesian criteria. For version (4.9) n must be fixed and then an approximate design must be considered, regardless the value of n. In what follows we assume the criteria for nonlinear models since the linear case can be considered as a particular case. With mild additional conditions allowing the permutation of the integral with the limit, the directional derivative can be computed in all cases as

$$\partial\Phi^B[M_B(\xi), M_B(\xi')] = \mathrm{E}_\theta \left\{\partial\Phi[M_B(\xi), M_B(\xi')]\right\},$$
$$\partial\Phi^{sB}[M(\xi), M(\xi')] = \mathrm{E}_\theta \left\{\partial\Phi[M(\xi), M(\xi')]\right\}.$$

In particular, for differentiable criteria, the directional derivatives are

$$\partial\Phi^B[M_B(\xi), M_B(\xi')] = \mathrm{E}_\theta \left(\mathrm{tr}\left\{\nabla\Phi[M_B(\xi)][M_B(\xi') - M_B(\xi)]\right\}\right),$$
$$\partial\Phi^{sB}[M(\xi), M(\xi')] = \mathrm{E}_\theta \left(\mathrm{tr}\left\{\nabla\Phi[M(\xi)][M(\xi') - M(\xi)]\right\}\right).$$

In all cases the known directional derivatives for the ordinary criteria can be used to compute all these Bayesian directional derivatives. Then the equivalence theorem can be stated as in Theorem 2.1 using these expressions.

4.4.1 D-optimality

The partial derivative is

$$\begin{aligned}
\partial \Phi_D^B[M_B(\xi), M_B(\xi_x)] &= \mathrm{E}_\theta \left(\mathrm{tr} \left\{ M_B^{-1}(\xi)[M_B(\xi_x) - M_B(\xi)] \right\} \right) \\
&= m - \mathrm{E}_\theta \left\{ \mathrm{tr} \left[M(\xi) + \frac{1}{n} R \right]^{-1} \left[f(x) f^T(x) + \frac{1}{n} R \right] \right\} \\
&= \mathrm{E}_\theta \left\{ \mathrm{tr}[M_B^{-1}(\xi) M(\xi)] - f^T(x) M_B^{-1}(\xi) f(x) \right\}, \\
\partial \Phi_D^{sB}[M(\xi), M(\xi_x)] &= m - f^T(x) \mathrm{E}_\theta [M^{-1}(\xi)] f(x).
\end{aligned}$$

This shows how both criteria are equivalent to the corresponding G-optimality criterion.

4.4.2 A-optimality

The partial derivative is

$$\begin{aligned}
\partial \Phi_A^B[M_B(\xi), M_B(\xi_x)] &= \mathrm{E}_\theta \left\{ \mathrm{tr}[M_B^{-1}(\xi) - M_B^{-2}(\xi) M_B(\xi_x)] \right\}, \\
\partial \Phi_A^{sB}[M(\xi), M(\xi_x)] &= \mathrm{E}_\theta \left\{ \mathrm{tr}[M^{-1}(\xi)] - f^T(x) \mathrm{E}_\theta [M^{-1}(\xi)] f(x) \right\}.
\end{aligned}$$

4.5 Examples

4.5.1 Simple Linear Regression

Let a simple linear regression model be

$$y = \theta_1 + \theta_2 x + \varepsilon, \ x \in [a, b],$$

with the usual assumptions of normality, homoscedasticity, and independence of the observations, and so the errors. The mean of the errors is assumed zero and the variance σ^2.

Let us assume a Gaussian prior distribution of the parameters with $\theta^{(0)} = (\theta_1^{(0)}, \theta_2^{(0)})^T$ and

$$R = \begin{pmatrix} r_1 & r_3 \\ r_3 & r_2 \end{pmatrix},$$

with $r_1 > 0$ and $r_1 r_2 - r_3^2 > 0$. Let us assume the optimal design is a two-extreme-point design,

$$\xi = \begin{Bmatrix} a & b \\ 1-p & p \end{Bmatrix}.$$

Then the determinant of the Bayesian Information Matrix is

$$\begin{aligned} \det M_B(\xi) &= \det\left[\begin{pmatrix} 1 & (1-p)a + pb \\ (1-p)a + pb & (1-p)a^2 + pb^2 \end{pmatrix} + \frac{1}{n}\begin{pmatrix} r_1 & r_3 \\ r_3 & r_2 \end{pmatrix}\right] \\ &= -(b-a)^2 p^2 + \beta p + \alpha, \end{aligned}$$

which is a parabola for some values of α and β independent of p, with the branches down with the maximum at the critical point $p_c = \frac{1}{2} + \frac{(b+a)r_1 - 2r_2}{2(b-a)n}$. Thus, the best among this design is for the weight

$$p^* = \begin{cases} p_c & \text{if } p_c \in [0, 1], \\ 0 & \text{if } p_c < 0, \\ 1 & \text{if } p_c > 1. \end{cases}$$

In particular,

$$p^* = \frac{1}{2}\left(1 + \frac{(a+b)r_1 - 2r_3}{n(b-a)}\right),$$

and $p_c \in [0, 1]$ if and only if $n \geq \frac{(a+b)r_1 - 2r_3}{b-a}$, that is, for n large enough the Bayesian optimal design jumps from one to two points. This is an interesting and extensible behavior valid for other models.

These are some particular cases using the same precision matrix for $r_1 = 2$, $r_2 = 1$, and $r_3 = 1$,

1. Let $a = -2$, $b = -1$, then $|((a+b)r_1 - 2r_3)/(b-a)| = 8$. Thus, $p^* = 0$ for $n \leq 8$ and $p^* = \frac{n-8}{2n}$ otherwise.
2. Let $a = -1/4$, $b = 1/4$, then $|((a+b)r_1 - 2r_3)/(b-a)| = 4$. Thus, $p^* = 0$ for $n \leq 4$ and $p^* = \frac{n-4}{2n}$ otherwise.
3. Let $a = 1$, $b = 100$, then $|((a+b)r_1 - 2r_3)/(b-a)| = 200/99$. Thus, $p^* = 1$ for $n \leq 3$ and $p^* = \frac{200+99n}{198n}$ otherwise.

4.5.2 A Nonlinear Model

Let the Michaelis–Menten model be

$$y = \frac{Vx}{x+K} + \varepsilon,\ x \in [0, bK] = [0, B].$$

Normality, homoscedasticity, and independence of the observations, errors with mean zero, and variance σ^2 are assumed here. Sometimes the design space is expressed in function of the nonlinear parameter K. There are mainly tow advantages, the main one is that this is rather usual in practice, typically $[0, 5K]$. The second is that the optimal designs have nicer expressions. An extensive search for optimal experimental designs for this model has been performed by López Fidalgo and Wong (2002) in one of the first papers finding D- and c-optimal designs and pseudo-optimal designs with more than two points. They gave a closed form of the D-optimal design,

$$\xi_D^\star = \left\{ \begin{array}{cc} \frac{b}{2+b}K & bK \\ 1/2 & 1/2 \end{array} \right\}.$$

For the Bayesian approach dealing with the parameters has to be done carefully and therefore $\chi = [0, B]$ will be assumed in what follows. Let us consider a Gaussian prior distribution of the parameters with mean $\theta^{(0)} = (K^{(0)}, V^{(0)})^T$ and

$$R = \begin{pmatrix} r_1 & r_3 \\ r_3 & r_2 \end{pmatrix}.$$

For simplicity we start computing Φ^{sB}-optimal designs. In particular,

$$\Phi^{sB}[M(\xi)] = -\mathrm{E}[\log\det M(\xi)].$$

From the results of López Fidalgo and Wong (2002), it is likely that the optimal design is a two-point design including the ending point of the interval, B. Thus, let us assume designs of the type

$$\xi = \left\{ \begin{array}{cc} A & B \\ 1-p & p \end{array} \right\}.$$

Then, after some algebra it can be seen that

$$\begin{aligned} \Phi^{sB}[M(\xi)] = -\mathrm{E}[&\log A^2B^2(B-A)^2 + \log p(1-p) + 2\log V \\ &-4\log(A+K) - 4\log(B+K)]]. \end{aligned}$$

As happens with ordinary D-optimality the weights must be equal. Using the second-order Taylor expansion with respect to the prior mean of the parameters, an approximate expression of the expectations can be obtained,

$$\mathrm{E}(\log V) \approx \log V_0 - \frac{r_1}{2V_0^2},$$

$$\mathrm{E}(\log(A+K)) \approx \log(A+K_0) - \frac{r_2}{2(A+K_0)^2}.$$

Thus, the objective function on A can be reduced to maximizing

$$\log A^2(B-A)^2 - 4\log(A+K_0) + \frac{2r_2}{(A+K_0)^2}.$$

For instance, if $K = 100,\ B = 5K,\ r_2 = 0.1$, then the Bayesian optimal design is

$$\xi = \left\{ \begin{matrix} 33.3 & 500 \\ 1/2 & 1/2 \end{matrix} \right\},$$

while the non-Bayesian D-optimal first point is $100\dot{5}/7 = 71.4$.

4.6 Exercises

Exercise 4.1 Compute D-optimal Bayesian designs for the model

$$y = \theta_0 \cos(x) + \theta_1 \sin(x) + \varepsilon,\ x \in \chi = [0, \pi/3],$$

assuming a Gaussian prior distribution of the parameters with

$$R = \begin{pmatrix} r_1 & r_3 \\ r_3 & r_2 \end{pmatrix},$$

for a general value of $n \geq 4$.

(a) $r_1 = 2,\ r_2 = 3,\ r_3 = 0.$
(b) $r_1 = 2,\ r_2 = 3,\ r_3 = 1.$

Solution

(a)

$$\left\{ \begin{matrix} 0 & \pi/3 \\ \frac{n+1}{2n} & \frac{n-1}{2n} \end{matrix} \right\}.$$

(b)

$$\left\{ \begin{matrix} 0 & \pi/3 \\ \frac{3(n+1)+2\sqrt{3}}{6n} & \frac{3(n-1)-2\sqrt{3}}{6n} \end{matrix} \right\}.$$

Exercise 4.2 Compute universal optimal pseudo-Bayesian designs for the model $y = e^{\theta x} + \varepsilon,\ x \in \chi = [a, b]$, assuming Gaussian prior distribution of the parameters with mean $\theta_0 > 0$.

Solution $\left\{ \begin{matrix} b \\ 1 \end{matrix} \right\}.$

Chapter 5
Hot Topics

5.1 Introduction

This chapter is devoted to particular topics of interest as well as recent developments in OED. Some of them are motivated from some of the criticisms considered in the first chapter. In particular, computer experiment, which is an emerging area becoming more and more popular, is introduced. Complex experiments, which are not practicable in real situations, are emulated with complex and slow computer experiments. Thus, a suitable optimal design is needed in this situation. First, a proper objective criterion function has to be introduced. Then efficient algorithms to compute the designs are crucial here. In the face of the recent "Big Data" phenomenon, the role of statistics is crucial in extracting maximum information from data, which is the motivation behind the design of experiments in what is called active learning (AL).

There is an innovative proposal of how Optimal Experimental Design can contribute to the important topic of personalized medicine. Designing for discriminating between models when there are several rival models before the data is collected is another modern topic in model selection. Different approaches are considered also for nonnormal models.

Frequently, in the real life some of the explanatory variables may be designed, but some other have values already known when designing and are not under the control of the experimenter. Sometimes, there is another kind of explanatory variable, which is not under the control of the experimenter, but its values are unknown before the experiment is realized. This situation is considered from the design point of view, which in the later case needs some prior assumptions. Three real examples are provided in Chap. 6.

The word "optimal" in the topic of this book means this theory needs efficient algorithms for computing optimal designs. Actually, this is not an easy task and deserves much work to be done in this direction. During years traditional algorithms in the area have been used without much ambition to get something better. Recently

J. López-Fidalgo, *Optimal Experimental Design*, Lecture Notes in Statistics 226,
https://doi.org/10.1007/978-3-031-35918-7_5

there is a good number of publications in this area, which is a good news. For instance, there is some attention on nature-inspired algorithms. They are simple to implement and produce good results in spite of convergence cannot be proved mathematically. A few simple examples of typical meta-heuristic algorithms will be shown in detail.

5.2 Computer Experiments

Experimental design is especially important in practice when an experiment is quite expensive or it is impossible to realize, for instance, due to ethical constraints or too long experiments. In some cases, a thoughtful mathematical study may lead to a complex system of differential equations simulating the procedure and the results. This deterministic model is called a *simulator* reproducing real experiments *in-silico*, also referred to *digital twins* simulating a real scenario or phenomenon. Changing the values of the variables, different results are obtained. An example could be developing an automated way of saving energy keeping a continuous comfortable temperature in a building. Variables such as the structure of the building, the exposure of the walls to the sun and the wind, the utilization of the different room along the day (and night), the weather forecasting, among other, and the thermostat, which is what they want to control, will be used to adjust the model. The variations in the interior temperature of the building will be used as response variable. There are actually some simulators to obtain these results.

Frequently solving such systems of equations is computationally very demanding, for example, needing supercomputers and much time to give a solution. This is very useful since the real experimentation is not needed, but it has still this limitation. Even if the time to get a result is not big there could be so many possible combinations of the possible values of the variables that the simulator experimenter could be lost selecting those looking like more informative. Let us stress again that these simulators are deterministic models. If one repeats the simulation with the same values of the variables, the results will be exactly the same. Thus, it seems there is not space for statistics here.

The idea of the parsimonious principle of statistics can be applied to this problem to help in an analogous way. A much simpler model can be substituted emulating the complex deterministic simulator. A model of such characteristics is sometimes called *emulator*. Of course, there is not only one possible emulator as always happens in statistical modeling. Moreover, for fitting this model, the response comes from the simulator without error. This is an important issue if we want to deal with the problem with our statistical methods. Of course, we can always fit the model with LSEs and use classical analyses, but uncertainty measures based on residuals have no clear statistical meaning. Goodness of fit cannot be assigned, but there may be some systematic bias. If the interest is in prediction, then there is some uncertainty, although not directly with the parameters.

For the experimental design, replicates, randomization, or blocking have no sense in this scenario. However, this is an experimental design problem anyway. Thus, just exact designs with no replicates should be used or else approximate designs constraint to have equal weights. This last approach needs to take into account that approximate designs are considered and compared always under the same sample size hypothesis. That is, an approximate design with two points in its support could be better than a three-point design, both with equal weights. This comparison applies for instance realizing 60 experiments in total, 30 and 30 for the first design and 20, 20, and 20 for the second. But if no replications are allowed, the second design with just three experiments could be better than the first one with only two experiments.

Usually, the complex differential equations system must be solved through an algorithm, for example, changing the initial values to start the search randomly using, for instance, discrete event simulation or finite element procedures. This can produce slightly different results and/or different computing times. Since time of computation is an important issue, it is sometimes considered in the model, for example, with some total time of computation limit. It is worth to mention that a simulator could be very poor with uncertain consequences. Another very important issue is the correlation between computer experiments. Assuming correlated observations has been considered in Chap. 3.10.

Explainability and *interpretability* of a black box model is one of the main issues in Data Science. Statistics and experimental design can help to do this job jointly with the typical machine learning procedures.

A common feature of these type of experiments is high dimensional inputs and multivariate response. It is well-known the complexity this adds to the experimental design theory.

The use of computer experiments started in the 1980s. Sacks et al. (1989) made a good synthesis of the problem by using a Bayesian point of view. Chen et al. (2009) made a more recent review and Fehr et al. (1990) considered the frequentist approach.

Taguchi (1986) proposed the distinction between control factors, say x_{con}, and noise factors, x_{noise}. Then using a loss function, $L(y)$, the problem of finding the most informative values of the variables under control is

$$\min_{x_{con}} \int L[y(x_{con}, x_{noise})]\Gamma(dx_{noise}),$$

where Γ is the probability distribution of the noise.

MUCM (Managing Uncertainty in Complex Models) was a research project (2006-2012) for dealing with issues of uncertainty in computer experiments. MUCM techniques address questions such as uncertainty quantification, uncertainty propagation, uncertainty analysis, sensitivity analysis, calibration (or tuning, history matching, etc.), and ensemble analysis. They developed the useful MUCM toolkit.

Let us consider the model for the response,

$$y(x) = f^T(x)\beta + \varepsilon(x),$$

where $\mathrm{E}[\varepsilon(x)] = 0$, $\mathrm{E}[\varepsilon(u) \cdot \varepsilon(v)] = \sigma^2 R(u, v)$. Let $\xi = \{x_1, \ldots, x_n\}$ be an exact design with different points, $Y_\xi = (y(x_1), \ldots, y(x_n))^T$ the corresponding responses and let $\hat{y}(x) = c^T(x) Y_\xi$ be a possible linear predictor, which can be of different types,

1. The *BLUP (Best Linear Unbiased Predictor)* comes from the optimization problem,

$$\min_{c(x)} \mathrm{MSE}[\hat{y}(x)] = \mathrm{E}[c^T(x) Y_\xi - y(x)], // \ s.t.\ \mathrm{E}[c^T(x) Y_\xi] = \mathrm{E}[y(x)] = f^T(x)\beta,$$

   where MSE stands for the Mean Squared Error.
2. A *Bayesian predictor* comes from the posterior mean,

$$\hat{y}(x) = \mathrm{E}[y(x) | Y_\xi].$$

   It is known that in the Gaussian case the limit of the Bayesian predictor when the variance of the parameters goes to zero is the BLUP.

   Let us be more specific,

$$F = \begin{pmatrix} f^T(x_1) \\ \cdots \\ f^T(x_n) \end{pmatrix}, \ R = \{R(x_i, x_j)\}_{ij}, \ r(x) = \begin{pmatrix} R(x_1, x) \\ \cdots \\ R(x_n, x) \end{pmatrix}.$$

Then

$$\mathrm{MSE}[\hat{y}(x)] = \sigma^2 [1 + c^T(x) R c(x) - 2 c^T(x) r(x)]$$
$$s.t. \mathrm{E}[c^T(x) Y_\xi] = F^T c(x) = f(x).$$

Using Lagrange multipliers the BLUP is obtained as follows:

$$\begin{pmatrix} 0 & F^T \\ F & R \end{pmatrix} \begin{pmatrix} \lambda(x) \\ c(x) \end{pmatrix} = \begin{pmatrix} f(x) \\ r(x) \end{pmatrix},$$

then

$$\hat{y}(x) = f^T(x)\hat{\beta} + r^T(x) R^{-1} (Y_\xi - F\hat{\beta}),$$

where

$$\hat{\beta} = (F^T R^{-1} F)^{-1} F^T R^{-1} Y_\xi.$$

Therefore,

$$\mathrm{MSE}[\hat{y}(x)] = \sigma^2 \left[1 - (f^T(x), r^T(x)) \begin{pmatrix} 0 & F^T \\ F & R \end{pmatrix} \begin{pmatrix} f(x) \\ r(x) \end{pmatrix} \right].$$

Remark 5.1

1. Typically

$$R(u, v) = R(|u - v|).$$

2. For a multivariate case,

$$R(u, v) = \prod_j R_j(|u_j - v_j|).$$

3. A typical case is the exponential.

$$R(u, v) = \prod_j \exp(-\theta_j |u_j - v_j|^p),\ 0 < p \leq 2.$$

For $p = 1$ we have the Ornstein-Uhlenbeck process.

4. Another usual case is the so-called linear spline,

$$R(u, v) = \prod_j (1 - \theta_j |u_j - v_j|)_+,$$

where

$$f_+(x) = \begin{cases} f(x) & \text{if } f(x) \geq 0, \\ 0 & \text{if } f(x) \leq 0. \end{cases}$$

5. Assuming a Gaussian process the MLE of σ^2 is

$$\hat{\sigma}^2 = \frac{1}{n}(Y_\xi - F\hat{\beta})^T R^{-1}(Y_\xi - F\hat{\beta}),$$

then the parameters of the covariance can be obtained minimizing $(\det R)^{1/n}\hat{\sigma}^2$.

6. A usual technique to estimate the covariance structure for lower dimension is Kriging. This consists basically in estimating the variogram $\mathrm{E}[\varepsilon(u) - \varepsilon(v)]^2$.

5.2.1 Design Criteria

Some criteria are based on the MSE matrix,

$$M = \mathrm{E}\left\{[Y(x_i) - \hat{y}(x_i)][Y(x_j) - \hat{y}(x_j)]\right\}_{i,j}.$$

These are typical criteria for computer experiments,

1. *Integrated Mean Squared Error* (IMSE):

$$\begin{aligned}\text{IMSE}(\xi) &= \int_\chi \text{MSE}[\hat{y}(x)]\mu(dx) \\ &= \sigma^2 \left\{1 - \text{tr}\left[\begin{pmatrix} 0 & F^T \\ F & R \end{pmatrix} \int \begin{pmatrix} f(x)f^T(x) & f(x)r^T(x) \\ r(x)f^T(x) & r(x)r^T(x) \end{pmatrix} \mu(dx)\right]\right\}\end{aligned}$$

   for some measure μ.
2. *Maximum Mean Squared Error* (MMSE).
3. *Entropy*: Let g be the conditional density of $Y(\cdot)$ on $\bar{\chi} = \chi - S_\xi$ given Y_ξ, where S_ξ is the support of ξ. The criterion consists in minimizing its entropy $\text{E}(-\log g)$. This is equivalent to minimizing the prior entropy on S_ξ. For a Gaussian process this means minimizing the determinant of the covariance matrix of $Y(\cdot)$ on ξ.

5.2.2 Including the Computation Time in the Model

The time of computation for each experiment could be of importance in some cases where the conditions of the experiment (values of the explanatory variables) could greatly increase the complexity of the computations. For this reason time is sometimes considered in the model. Let τ be time of the computer experiment (simulation) for $x \in \chi$ and consider the model for the response,

$$y(x, \tau) = f^T(x)\beta + z(x) + \varepsilon(x, \tau),$$

where $\text{E}[\varepsilon(x, \tau)] = 0$, $\text{E}[\varepsilon(u, \tau_u) \cdot \varepsilon(v, \tau_v)] = 0$, $\text{var}[\varepsilon(x, \tau)] = \frac{\sigma^2}{\omega(\tau)}$, $\text{E}[z(x)] = 0$, $\text{E}[z(u) \cdot z(v)] = \sigma_z^2 c(u, v)$, $\text{var}[z(x)] = \sigma_z^2$, and ε and z are independent. Let $\eta(x) = f^T(x)\beta + z(x)$.

Let $\xi = \{x_i, \tau_i\}_{i=1}^n$ be an exact design such that $\sum_{i=1}^n \tau_i = T$ for predetermined values of T and n. A Gaussian process is assumed,

$$Y(\xi) \sim \mathcal{N}\left(F^T\beta, \sigma_z^2\Sigma_Y\right),$$

where $F^T = (f(x_1), \ldots, f(x_n))$, $\sigma_z^2\Sigma_Y = \sigma_z^2 C + \sigma^2\text{diag}[\omega(x)]$, and C is the matrix built with function c.

The BLUE estimator is then

$$\hat{\beta} = (F\Sigma_Y^{-1}F^T)^{-1}F\Sigma_Y^{-1}Y(\xi), \;\; \Sigma_{\hat{\beta}} = \sigma_z^2(F\Sigma_Y^{-1}F^T)^{-1}.$$

The Best Linear Unbiased Predictor (BLUP) is

$$\hat{\eta}(x|\xi) = f^T(x)\hat{\beta} + c^T(x)\Sigma_{\hat{\beta}}^{-1}[Y(\xi) - F^T\hat{\beta}],\ \Sigma_{\hat{\beta}} = \sigma_z^2(F\Sigma_Y^{-1}F^T)^{-1},$$

coming from the optimization problem

$$\min_{\hat{Y}=\sum_i c_i Y_i} \text{var}[\eta(\xi) - \hat{Y}],\ \text{s.t. var}[\eta(\xi) - \hat{Y}] = 0,$$

where $c(x) = (c(x, x_1), \ldots, c(x, x_n))^T$.

And the Mean Squared Prediction Error (MSPE) is then

$$\begin{aligned}\rho(x) &= \mathrm{E}\{[\hat{\eta}(x|\xi) - \eta(x)]^2\}\\ &= \sigma_z\{1 - c^T(x)\Sigma_Y^{-1}c(x) + [f(x) - F\Sigma_Y^{-1}c(x)]^T(F\Sigma_Y^{-1}F^T)^{-1}[f(x)\\ &\quad -F\Sigma_Y^{-1}c(x)]\}\\ &= \sigma_z[1 - c^T(x)\Sigma_Y^{-1}c(x)].\end{aligned}$$

The optimality criterion will be the Integrated Mean Squared Error (IMSE),

$$\text{IMSE}(\xi) = \int_\chi \rho(x)\mu(dx)$$

for an appropriate measure μ. Similarly other distance-based criteria can be used in the same way.

5.3 Active Learning

As mentioned repeatedly in this book the aim of experimental design theory is to find a good (optimal if possible) experimental design to save experiments and reduce the number of experiments as much as possible. In the era of Big Data and the easy to obtain more data than we are able to process and analyze, the area of experimental design seems to be old-fashioned or at least very much restricted to some critical experiments such as clinical trials. The objective of the optimization of a plan of experimentation is to do good inferences. For that the covariance matrix of the estimates of the parameters plays an essential role, although there are some optimality criteria not based on it. Actually, the main goal is to detect the most informative experiments.

Instead of talking about Big Data frequently, we should refer to big computing since the main problem is to do computations for a statistical analysis with a huge number of data. A typical technique to deal with this is to do sub-sampling from the big sample. As a matter of fact, this is what statisticians have been doing for years. The news here is that in the classical approach the sample is obtained from the whole population while frequently here the (sub)sample is withdrawn from a huge sample. If both samples are representative of the population everything works. Since the main idea of optimal experimental design is to detect the points with more information, this idea could be used here to address the sampling to the most informative parts of the big sample. This is currently called *active learning* (AL) while the simple random sampling (SRS) is called *passive learning* (PL).

In this context we may have several possible scenarios:

1. The big sample contains values from both, the explanatory variables and the responses.
2. The big sample contains just values of the explanatory variables. Then the responses will be observed just for the subsample. This may happen when observing the responses requires expensive and complicated procedures, such as a genetic PCR.
3. The big sample contains values of some explanatory variables and/or the responses. This scenario includes actually several different situations.

Let $\mathcal{Q}$ be the Big Data sample. Assume χ is the set of different values of the p explanatory variables and assume the size of $\mathcal{Q}$ is N. The response y is modeled through a pdf $h(y|x,\theta)$ as usual. The objective is to find a sampling probability distribution $\{\pi_i\}_i^N$ to do weighted subsampling and obtain a subsample $(x_i^\star, y_i^\star)$, $i = 1, \ldots, n$. Here the y_i may have been observed before or after the sampling as mentioned above. Frequently these weights are based on normalized statistical leverage scores (*algorithmic leveraging*).

There are two possible scenarios in the Big Data world,

1. The so-called *high dimensional data* $p >> N$. Tibshirani (1996) provided the popular LASSO for data dimension reduction.
2. More recent is the situation of $p << N$ with a huge amount of subjects.

Coming back to the big computing problem, it is worth to mention that for Ordinary Least Squares in linear regression fitting the computing time is $O(Np^2)$. This offers a reference showing how much "worse" is having a big p than a big N. Wang et al. (2019) proved that "intelligent" sub-sampling may reduce this complexity to $O(np)$. In what follows the linear model is considered to see how active learning works.

For the linear regression model the number of parameters is $m = p+1$, including the intercept. Let X be the full $N \times (p+1)$ design matrix, including a first column of one's, and Y the full $N \times 1$ vector of responses using all the data. Then the LSEs are $\hat{\theta} = (X^T X)^{-1} X^T Y$ and the information matrix is $M = \frac{1}{\sigma^2}(X^T X)^{-1}$. Let $X^\star$ be the subsample $n \times (p+1)$ design matrix and $Y^\star$ the sample $n \times 1$ vector of responses. Then the LSEs are $\hat{\theta}^\star = (X^{\star T} X^\star)^{-1} X^{\star T} Y^\star$ and the information matrix is $M^\star = \frac{1}{\sigma^2}(X^{\star T} X^\star)^{-1}$. The sampling scheme is defined by an indicator function,

$$\delta_i = \begin{cases} 1 \text{ if } (x_i^\star, y_i^\star) \text{ is in the sample,} \\ 0 \text{ if } (x_i^\star, y_i^\star) \text{ is not in the sample,} \end{cases} \quad i = 1, \ldots, N.$$

The optimal sampling will be made according to some criterion.

$$\delta^{\star} = \arg\min_{\delta} \Phi[M(\delta)], \text{ where } \sum_{i=1}^{N} \delta_i = n.$$

This has a parallelism with optimal experimental design. This indicator defines a probability distribution on χ in a straightforward way, say ξ. Thus, there are three probability distributions very much related. On the one hand, $\{\pi_i\}_i^N$ is the prior subsampling distribution and either $\{\delta_i\}_i^N$ or ξ is the actual probability distribution of the obtained sample. Now there is not a simple random sampling (SRS) and therefore the estimators need some correction, weighting accordingly the sample points,

$$\tilde{\theta} = \left(\sum_{i=1}^{N} \omega_i n_i x_i x_i^T\right)^{-1} \sum_{i=1}^{N} \omega_i n_i x_i y_i,$$

where x_i is the i-th column of X^T and n_i is the number of times it appears in the sample.

These are typical distributions for π and ω,

(i) *Uniform:* $\pi_i = \frac{1}{N}$ and $\omega_i = 1$.
(ii) *Leverage-based sampling:* $\pi_i = \frac{h_{ii}}{p+1}$ and $\omega_i = \frac{1}{\pi_i}$, where $h_{ii} = x_i^T (X^T X)^{-1} x_i$.
(iii) *Shrinked leveraging sampling:* $\pi_i = \frac{\alpha h_{ii}}{p+1} + \frac{1-\alpha}{N}$ and $\omega_i = \frac{1}{\pi_i}$.

Usually $\omega_i = 1/\pi_i$ to undo the weighing in the sampling step or just unweighted $\omega_i = 1$ giving actually more weight to the selected more informative points. Another possibility is to optimize these weights as well according to some criterion.

If the sampling is assumed with replacement, then $n_i \sim \mathcal{B}(N, \pi_i)$. Let us define

$$M = \mathrm{E}[M(\xi)|X] = \frac{1}{\sigma^2} \sum_{i=1}^{N} \mathrm{E}(n_i) x_i x_i^T = \frac{N}{\sigma^2} \sum_{i=1}^{N} \pi_i x_i x_i^T.$$

Theorem 5.1 *Let* $\Delta = \{\xi \mid \sum_{i=1}^{N} n_i x_i x_i^T$ *nonsingular*$\}$ *and the indicator* $I_\Delta(\xi) = 1$ *if* $\xi \in \Delta$. *If* $I_\Delta(\xi) = 1$, *then* $\tilde{\theta}$ *is unbiased and*

$$\Sigma_{\{\tilde{\theta} \mid X, I_\Delta(\xi)=1\}} \geq P[I_\Delta(\xi) = 1 \mid X] M^{-1} = \frac{\sigma^2 P[I_\Delta(\xi) = 1 \mid X]}{N} \left\{\sum_{i=1}^{N} \pi_i x_i x_i^T\right\}^{-1}.$$

The proof can be found in Wang et al. (2019).

Remark 5.2 If $N >> p$ then $\mathrm{P}[I_\Delta(\xi) = 1 \mid X] \approx 1$.

Applying this result to the three particular cases given above and assuming a sample size of n,

(i) *Uniform sampling:*

$$\Sigma_{\{\tilde{\theta}_{UNIF}\,|\,X,\,I_\Delta(\xi)=1\}} \geq \frac{\sigma^2 \mathrm{P}[I_\Delta(\xi)=1\,|\,X]}{n}\left(\frac{1}{N}\sum_{i=1}^{N} x_i x_i^T\right)^{-1}$$

$$\longrightarrow_{n\to\infty} \frac{\sigma^2 \mathrm{P}[I_\Delta(\xi)=1\,|\,X]}{n}[\mathrm{E}(xx^T)]^{-1}.$$

(ii) *Leverage-based sampling:*

$$\Sigma_{\{\tilde{\theta}_{LEV}\,|\,X,\,I_\Delta(\xi)=1\}} \geq \frac{\sigma^2 (p+1)\mathrm{P}[I_\Delta(\xi)=1\,|\,X]}{n} \times \left(\sum_{i=1}^{N} x_i x_i^T (X^T X)^{-1} x_i x_i^T\right)^{-1}$$

$$\longrightarrow_{n\to\infty} \frac{\sigma^2 (p+1)\mathrm{P}[I_\Delta(\xi)=1\,|\,X]}{n} \times \left(\mathrm{E}\left\{xx^T[\mathrm{E}(xx^T)]^{-1}xx^T\right\}\right)^{-1}.$$

(iii) *Shrieked leveraging sampling:*

$$\Sigma_{\{\tilde{\theta}_{SLEV}\,|\,X,\,I_\Delta(\xi)=1\}} \geq \frac{\sigma^2 (p+1)\mathrm{P}[I_\Delta(\xi)=1\,|\,X]}{n} \times \left(\frac{\alpha}{p+1}\sum_{i=1}^{N} x_i x_i^T (X^T X)^{-1} x_i x_i^T + \frac{1-\alpha}{N}\sum_{i=1}^{N} x_i x_i^T\right)^{-1}$$

$$\longrightarrow_{n\to\infty} \frac{\sigma^2 \mathrm{P}[I_\Delta(\xi)=1\,|\,X]}{n} \times \left(\frac{\alpha}{p+1}\mathrm{E}\{xx^T[\mathrm{E}(xx^T)]^{-1}xx^T + (1-\alpha)\mathrm{E}(xx^T)\}\right)^{-1}.$$

Remark 5.3 Using a more compact notation let $W = \mathrm{diag}\{\omega_1, \ldots, \omega_n\}$. The weighted estimator is then

$$\tilde{\theta} = (X^T W X)^{-1} X^T W Y$$

and the covariance matrix of these estimators for uncorrelated observations, $\Sigma_Y = \sigma^2 I$, is

$$\Sigma_{\tilde{\theta}} = \sigma^2 (X^T W X)^{-1} X^T W^2 X (X^T W X)^{-1}.$$

If the weights were all equal, then we obtain the usual covariance matrix for uncorrelated observations,

$$\Sigma_{\tilde{\theta}} = \sigma^2 (X^T X)^{-1}.$$

Example 5.1

1. **Linear model:** A typical linear model with two variables is considered here,

$$y = \theta_1 + \theta_2 x + \theta_3 z + \varepsilon,\ \varepsilon \sim \mathcal{N}(0, \sigma^2)$$

We simulate 10^5 values of two normal explanatory variables with means 1 and 3, respectively, and standard deviations 3 and 2. The error was simulated with another normal distribution with mean 0 and standard deviation 10. Then values of the response are computed using these coefficient values,

$$y = 1 + 2x - z + \varepsilon,\ \varepsilon \sim \mathcal{N}(0, \sigma^2)$$

Assuming a compact design space $\chi = [a, b] \times [c, d]$, the D-optimal design for this model is equally supported at the vertices of the rectangle (Wang et al., 2019),

$$\xi_D^\star = \left\{ \begin{array}{cccc} (a, c) & (a, d) & (b, c) & (b, d) \\ 1/4 & 1/4 & 1/4 & 1/4 \end{array} \right\}.$$

But the potential points for the optimal design have to be chosen in the actual set of points given by the big sample we already have. Wang et al. (2019) proposed the following algorithm to get D-optimal subsampling,

(a) Assuming $r = n/2p$ is an integer (in this example $r = 100/4 = 20$), choose the r pairs with the smallest first component values and r with the largest.
(b) Excluding the $2r$ points selected in 1. choose the r pairs with the smallest second component values and r with the largest.
(c) Let $X_D^\star$ be the design matrix and $y_D^\star$ the corresponding responses of these $4r = 100$ points and compute the estimate $\theta_D^\star = [(X_D^\star)^T X_D^\star]^{-1} (X_D^\star)^T y_D^\star$ with the covariance matrix $\sigma[(X_D^\star)^T X_D^\star]^{-1}$.

Performing passive learning, leverage-based active learning with and without weighting for the fitting, and the D-optimal-based active learning, Table 5.1 displays the Mean Square Errors (MSE) using the whole dataset to compute them and not only the subsamples chosen. All the subsamples were of size 100. In the

Table 5.1 MSE for different subsampling with standard deviation between brackets

Whole	Passive (SRS)	Leverage (unweighted)	Leverage (weighted)	D-optimal
99.7	103.0 (2.95)	102.0 (1.95)	108.7 (2.34)	100.1

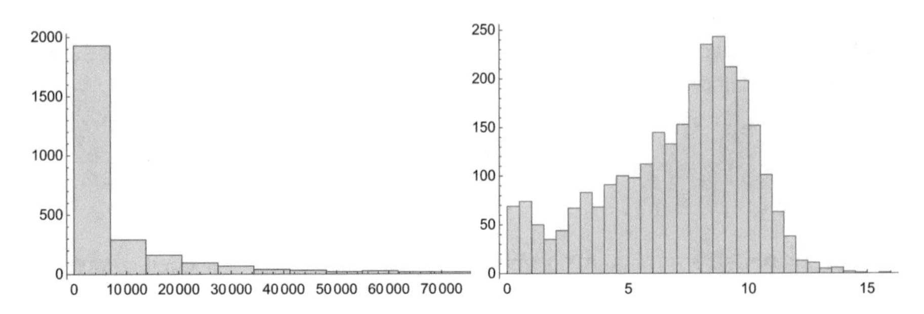

Fig. 5.1 Histograms of x_4 (left) and $\log(x_4 + 1)$ (right)

passive and active learning, it was repeated 20 times, so the mean of the MSEs is displayed with the standard deviation between brackets. D-optimality is the best by far. Then leverage-based active learning is slightly better than passive learning if no weights are considered for estimation.

2. **Classification:** Consider a toy (from a Big Data point of view), but real example of 1797 tweets. We are interested in detecting whether a tweet comes from a human or from a bot according to the explanatory variables provided by twitter: "friends," "listed," "favourites," "status," and "profile." The final variable is binary while the rest are counts. We assume that observing the label is expensive and laborious, so we are interested in doing "intelligent" subsampling to obtain maximum information with lower cost. For the classification a logistic model is being used,

$$P(y = 1 \mid \theta, x) = \frac{1}{1 + e^{-\theta^T x}}, \tag{5.1}$$

where $y = 1$ means the tweet comes from a bot and $y = 0$ from a human.

The first four variables are rather skewed (Fig. 5.1 shows the histogram of x_4 and $\log(x_4 + 1)$). Table 5.3 shows some indicators of the fitting where the *cut-off* for the probability classifying as bot or human was chosen for maximizing the *accuracy* (ratio of right classification). The second row shows the results for the logistic regression with the whole dataset. Using a logarithmic transformation $\log(x_i + 1), i = 1, 2, 3, 4$, much better results are obtained (see Table 5.3). Thus, all the subsampling will be preformed with this transformed dataset.

For simplicity, leverage-based sampling for a logistic model is being used here $\pi_i = \frac{h_{ii}}{p+1}$ and weights $\omega_i = \frac{1}{\pi_i}$ for fitting the logistic model, where $h_{ii} = \lambda_i x_i^T (X^T \Lambda X)^{-1} x_i$, $i = 1, \ldots, p+1$, and

$$\lambda_i = \frac{e^{-\theta^T x_i}}{(1 + e^{-\theta^T x_i})^2}, \quad \Lambda = \text{diag}\{\lambda_1, \ldots, \lambda_n\}.$$

Performing passive learning, leverage-based active learning with and without weighting for the fitting, and D-optimal-based active learning, Table 5.3 displays the maximum accuracy with its corresponding cut-off for the estimated probabilities to predict the label, the *area under the curve* (AUC), and the MSE using the whole dataset to compute them and not only the subsamples chosen. All the subsamples were of size 100, but the marginal D-optimal design, which will be explained later. In the passive and leverage-based active learning, it was repeated 20 times, so the mean of the MSEs is displayed with the standard deviation between brackets.

A marginal D-optimal design was computed for each of the five variables assuming design spaces as continuous intervals with extremes in the minimum and maximum values of the big sample for the first four variables and {0, 1} for the fifth one. The D-optimal designs obtained were two-point designs with equal masses (Table 5.2). Nominal values come from adjusting different logistic models to the whole dataset for each particular variable. Then the 32 possible combinations of the marginal optimal points were considered and the 3 nearer points to each one were selected using the Euclidean distance. Thus, 96 points were used, a bit less than the 100 points in the rest of the subsamples. We called this "marginal D-optimal design."

An approximate design with 97.2% D-efficiency for 100 steps, including the first 100 points added in the process, was obtained now using Wynn–Fedorov algorithm assuming the big sample as design space and allowing replicates of the same point. Finally, an almost optimal design with 99.97% efficiency was obtained using a coordinate descent algorithm allowing replicates of the same point. They produce good accuracy although other measures were better for leverage-based AL.

Table 5.2 Marginal D-optimal designs

	Nominal values				
Variable	Intercept	Slope	Design space	Optimal support points	
x_1	2.04	−0.47	[[0, 14.6]]	1.06	7.62
x_2	0.80	−0.28	[0, 13.4]	0	8.37
x_3	1.30	−0.41	[0, 13.5]	0	6.94
x_4	0.38	−0.07	[0, 17.7]	0	15.07
x_5	0.90	1.74	{0, 1}	0	1

Wynn–Fedorov algorithm is applied here as follows:

Step 0: Let ξ_0 be a nonsingular initial design;
Step $(s+1)$**a:** At Step s a design ξ_s is obtained, then compute

$$x_s = \arg\max_x \lambda(x) x^T M^{-1}(\xi_s) x;$$

Step $(s+1)$**b:** Compute $\xi_{s+1} = \frac{s+1}{s+2}\xi_s + \frac{1}{s+2}\xi_{x_s}$;
Stopping rule: Stop the algorithm when the bound δ for the efficiency will be overtaken,

$$\frac{m}{\lambda(x_s) x_s^T M^{-1}(\xi_s) x_s} \geq \delta.$$

It is worth mentioning that all sampling has been done with replications. But the meaning of replication is not the same as the usual concept in experimental design where one replicates the experiment in the same conditions obtaining similar, but not necessarily equal results. In this example the subjects are there with their conditions from the beginning. Replicating means using the same subject with the same label more than once for the fitting. The practical meaning of this is performing weighted fitting of the model. The more replications mean the less data we are using for the fitting. The results with the D-optimal designs are slightly better with just a few points considered. Nevertheless, the cut-off is extremely near 1, although this does not mean an "overclassification" of ones. The cause of this may be that D-optimal designs are usually quite extreme producing unbalanced probabilities for the groups (Table 5.3). Table 5.4 shows more clear differences for a sample size of 32.

Table 5.3 Fitting indicators for different subsampling schemes with standard deviation between brackets for a sample size of 100

Sampling	Accuracy	Cut-off	AUC	MSE
Raw data	0.757	0.406	0.845	0.168
Log data	0.812	0.976	0.883	0.138
PL	0.791 (0.017)	0.784 (0.034)	0.867 (0.012)	0.151 (0.011)
Leverage AL (unweighted)	0.806 (0.012)	0.520 (0.089)	0.874 (0.006)	0.144 (0.004)
Leverage AL (weighted)	0.795 (0.014)	0.452 (0.093)	0.869 (0.011)	0.150 (0.007)
D-optimal (marginal)	0.807	0.682	0.858	0.158
D-optimal (100)	0.812	1.000	0.880	0.187
D-optimal (approximate)	0.803	1.000	0.877	0.198

Table 5.4 Fitting indicators for different subsampling schemes with standard deviation between brackets for a sample size of 32

Sampling	Accuracy	Cut-off	AUC	MSE
Raw data	0.757	0.406	0.845	0.168
Log data	0.812	0.976	0.883	0.138
PL	0.766 (0.041)	0.729 (0.172)	0.832 (0.0430)	0.190 (0.035)
Leverage AL (unweighted)	0.787 (0.0257)	0.433 (0.169)	0.854 (0.0195)	0.169 (0.015)
Leverage AL (weighted)	0.789 (0.026)	0.534 (0.209)	0.855 (0.023)	0.168 (0.019)
D-optimal (marginal)	0.804	0.043	0.856	0.159
D-optimal (32)	0.810	1.000	0.878	0.180
D-optimal (approximate)	0.810	1.000	0.878	0.180

5.4 Personalized Medicine

The *efficacy* of a treatment to cure a disease has to be balanced against the side effects (*toxicity*) in the patient. Using general limits and a general treatment for all may be beneficial for a percentage of them, but not for most of them or all. For this reason, finding an optimal treatment for each patient is of great importance. This belongs to the field of personalized medicine. For this, it is necessary to model the evolution of the disease, for example, a tumor growth, according to the different factors related to the type of disease and also to the characteristics of the patient. This is what will allow establishing an efficient and minimally invasive therapy. Treatment over time would be a frequent scenario. Some models are not given explicitly but through differential equations that do not have a simple analytical solution. From a statistical point of view the process should be as follows:

1. Search for parsimonious models that are good enough.
2. Look for optimal experimental designs using criteria focused on reaching a target with the treatment chosen for a specific patient.
3. Perform the experiments and fit the model with the data.
4. Use the model to elaborate protocols or better user-friendly software for researchers, clinical professionals, and even patients.

5.4.1 Static Planning of the Treatment

This is the most simple case. In this scenario a complete and closed treatment is decided for a specific patient before starting the treatment. This is actually the case in a typical nonpersonalized situation. There is a response variable, y, in charge of assessing the actual improvement of the treatment. A measurement at the end of a treatment x, such as the dose, will be considered here. Explanatory variables are measured before the choice of treatment, say z, relative to a specific patient, such as age, sex, tumor size, hypertension, body mass index (BMI). If the response is quantitative, the objective will usually be something like keeping $y \leq c$, for a threshold c indicating healthy standards below it.

Consider a statistical model given by a parametric family of pdfs as usual,

$$\{h(y \mid z, x; \theta) \mid \theta = (\tau^T, \beta^T)^T \in \Theta\},$$

where z may include the intercept. Once the model is fitted and a particular patient arrives with a specific value of z, then a value of x has to be chosen to get $y \leq c$. The value of y is unknown so far and the model will be used for making this decision. This can be done using two different but frequently equivalent procedures.

1. We may ask the expected value of y be under c_1, to be safer,

$$\mathrm{E}(y \mid z, x; \theta) \equiv \eta(z, x; \theta) \leq c_1.$$

   If x is a scalar, then working x out of the inequality we may have something like $x \geq \mu_1(c_1, z; \theta)$ and thus the treatment to be applied will be $x = \mu_1(c_1, z; \theta)$.
2. Another way of choosing x may be based on the probability of reaching the threshold,

$$\mathrm{P}(y \leq c_2 \mid z, x; \theta) \geq \gamma.$$

   In this case a value for γ, such as 0.99, should be chosen in advance. If this probability is a function of x only through the mean, say $\eta(z, x; \theta)$, then it is equivalent to the previous approach. Otherwise x has to be worked out from the inequality obtaining something similar, for the one-dimensional case, for example, $x \geq \mu_2(c_2, \gamma, z; \theta)$ and so $x = \mu_2(c_2, \gamma, z; \theta)$ will be the treatment.

There is another model we can consider for this purpose. Since we only need the model to predict $y \leq c_2$, then a dichotomized variable can be used instead and a generalized linear model can be fitted, for instance, a logistic or a probit model,

$$\mathrm{P}(y \leq c_3 \mid z, x; \theta) = F\left[\theta^T (z^T, x^T)^T \mid c_3\right],$$

with a cumulative distribution function (cdf) F and then a cut-off γ for this probability has to be chosen in such a way

$$F(\theta^T (z^T, x^T)^T \mid c_3) \geq \gamma.$$

Again working x out the optimal treatment is obtained, $\hat{x} = \mu_3(c_3, \gamma, z; \hat{\theta})$.

In all these cases the optimal design criterion must focus on estimating μ_i, $i = 1, 2, 3$ optimally. The variance of the likelihood estimator of this quantity can be approximated by $c_z^T M^{-1} c_z$, where M is the information matrix and

$$c_z = \frac{\partial \mu_i}{\partial \theta}.$$

This is the usual c-optimality providing nominal values to the parameters as needed. Each value of z gives then a different optimal design, that is, a personalized optimal design for those patients with that value. Solving this problem is not that easy, the application of the optimal design theory here requires a particular approach since in the model there is a mixture of controllable ("designable") variables, x, and variables whose values will be known before planning the experiment, z. Actually, an empirical distribution is given by the random sample of patients, although a theoretical distribution could also be assumed for those variables. Sections 6.4, 6.5, 6.6 consider this approach with some examples (Cook & Thibodeau, 1980).

It is important to mention that the optimal experimental design is focused on obtaining a good estimator but not necessarily to get the best treatment for the patients entering the experiment. Thus, the ethical component has to be included in the design of the experiment.

Example 5.2

1. Let us consider a linear model,

$$y = \tau^T z + \beta x + \varepsilon, \ \varepsilon \sim \mathcal{N}(0, \sigma^2).$$

   Thus,

$$\mathrm{E}(y) = \tau^T z + \beta x \le c_1$$

   if

$$x \le \frac{c_1 - \tau^T z}{\beta} \equiv \mu_1(c_1, z; \theta),$$

   Where c_1 is a threshold we do not want to overcome. Therefore, the directional vector for c-optimality is then

$$c_z^T = \left(-\frac{1}{\beta} z^T, -\frac{c_1 - \tau^T z}{\beta^2}\right).$$

2. For the same linear model,

$$\gamma \le P(y \le c_2) = P\left(\mathcal{N}(0,1) \le \frac{c_2 - \beta x - \tau^T z}{\sigma}\right) = \Phi\left(\frac{c_2 - \beta x - \tau^T z}{\sigma}\right),$$

   that is,

$$z_\gamma \le \frac{c_2 - \beta x - \tau^T z}{\sigma},$$

where z_γ is the γ-quantile of the standard normal distribution and therefore

$$x \leq \frac{c_2 - \tau^T z + \sigma z_\gamma}{\beta} \equiv \mu_2(c_2, \gamma, z; \theta).$$

Therefore, the directional vector for c-optimality is then

$$c_z^T = \left(-\frac{1}{\beta} z^T, -\frac{c_2 + \sigma z_\gamma - \tau^T z}{\beta^2}\right).$$

3. Let us consider a logistic model according to previous considerations,

$$\mathrm{P}(y \leq c_3 \mid z, x; \theta) = \frac{1}{1 + e^{-\theta^T (z^T, x^T)^T}} \geq \gamma.$$

After some algebra, assuming x one-dimensional,

$$x \leq \frac{\log\left(\frac{1}{\gamma} - 1\right) - \tau^T z}{\beta} \equiv \mu_3(c_3, \gamma, z; \theta).$$

Therefore, the directional vector for c-optimality is then

$$c_z^T = \left(-\frac{1}{\beta} z^T, -\frac{\log\left(\frac{1}{\gamma} - 1\right) - \tau^T z}{\beta^2}\right).$$

The three functions μ_i to be estimated aim the same objective. Actually, first and second are equivalent if $c_1 = \sigma z_\gamma + c_2$; first and third are equivalent if $c_1 = \log\left(\frac{1}{\gamma} - 1\right)$; and second and third are equivalent if $c_2 = \log\left(\frac{1}{\gamma} - 1\right) - \sigma z_\gamma$.

As mentioned above the problem from this point is not so simple. In order to see how this process works, a simple regression model is considered,

$$y = \tau_0 + \tau_1 z + \beta x + \varepsilon,\ z, x \in \{0, 1\},\ \varepsilon \sim \mathcal{N}(0, \sigma^2).$$

Assume the values of z come from a Bernoulli distribution of parameter 1/3. This distribution usually comes from the population of patients. The aim is to find optimal conditional designs of the type.

$$\xi(\cdot|z = 0) = \left\{\begin{matrix} 0 & 1 \\ 1 - p & p \end{matrix}\right\},\ \xi(\cdot|z = 1) = \left\{\begin{matrix} 0 & 1 \\ 1 - q & q \end{matrix}\right\}.$$

The FIM should include the whole model where x is “designable” and z is given,

$$\begin{pmatrix} 1 & z & x \\ z & z^2 & zx \\ x & xz & x^2 \end{pmatrix}.$$

Taking into account the “empirical” distribution of z, say ξ_z, and the general form of the conditional designs a general join design is of the type,

$$\xi(\cdot,\cdot) = \xi_z(\cdot)\xi(\cdot|\cdot) = \begin{Bmatrix} (0,0) & (0,1) & (1,0) & (1,1) \\ 2(1-p)/3 & 2p/3 & (1-q)/3 & q/3 \end{Bmatrix}.$$

This the most general FIM, restricted to the marginal distribution, is

$$\frac{1}{3}\begin{pmatrix} 3 & 1 & 2p+q \\ 1 & 1 & q \\ 2p+q & q & 2p+q \end{pmatrix}.$$

The vector coming from 1. is

$$c_z^T = \left(-\frac{1}{\beta}z^T, -\frac{c_1 - \tau^T z}{\beta^2}\right).$$

Assuming nominal values of the parameters $\tau_0 = \tau_1 = \beta = 1$ and $c_1 = 2$. Thus, $c_z^T = (-1, -z, z-1)$. After some algebra,

$$c_z^T M^{-1} c_z = \begin{cases} \frac{-6p+3(2-q)(1+q)}{4(1-p)p+2(1-q)q} & \text{if } z = 0 \\ \frac{6(1-p)p+3q}{2(1-p)p+(1-q)q} & \text{if } z = 1 \end{cases}.$$

For $z = 0$ there optimal weights minimizing this is $p^\star = 1$ for any value of q, while for $z = 1$ the optimal is reached for $q^\star = 0$ and any value of p. This means that for all patients with $z = 0$ all the experiments will be realized at $x = 1$, while for all patients with $z = 1$ all the experiments will be realized at $x = 0$. This is not an exciting result since this is a toy example for showing the procedure.

5.4.2 *Dynamic Planning of the Treatment*

Let us illustrate this with an example. Consider patients with a particular cancer. There is a general protocol for all of them consisting in receiving a particular type of chemotherapy in a first stage. The choice of this treatment has usually to do with efficacy but also with costs for the public health system and also with the severity of the side effects of the drug for the patients. Some not-easy-to-do analyses are performed to the patient at established times to check whether the treatment is

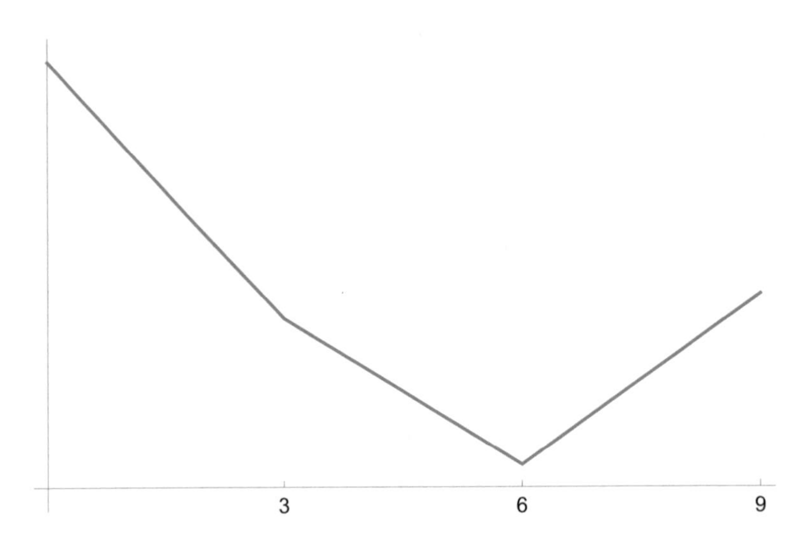

Fig. 5.2 Measurements of a bio-marker of a tumor during the treatment

effective. This will inform, for example, whether the treatment has become resistant, and some other treatment needs to be tried as soon as possible. In this process a number of things can be personalized to a particular patient, such as the doses and the times to be administered, as well as the type of drug chosen in a first stage. Just for this example we can consider personalizing the times to perform the analyses. This is very important since a quick detection of the resistance to the treatment will inform a new drug in a second stage needs to be tried as soon as possible. Thus, for a particular patient with a particular age, sex, size of tumor, and dose, a specific time will be assigned for the next analysis. A situation as the one described in Fig. 5.2 can be avoided in benefit of the patient but also the public health system. The behavior of the tumor is analyzed every three weeks, which it is estimated a right period for most of the cases. Personalizing this to the individual with all his or her features at the time of each analysis may save lives.

In this case the model describing the progress of the disease is longitudinal and a structure of correlation has to be considered. Some models of this type with correlated observations have been considered above. The outline of the problem is similar to the one considered in the last section, taking into account the novelty of the longitudinal feature.

5.5 Model Selection: Discrimination Between Rival Models

The ideas of this section come partially from López-Fidalgo and Tommasi (2018). One of the main criticisms to OED is that a design has to be found for a particular model and the model has to be guessed without having the data yet. Honestly speaking, we should say there are not solutions to this issue, which in fact is still present even with the data at hand. George Box used to say that "Models, of course, are never true, but fortunately it is only necessary that they be useful," for example, Box (1979). In a variety of situations before having the data, two or more models may be potential candidates. In the era of Big Data, model selection has become a hot topic, and so finding optimal experimental designs for that is crucial. From the point of view of the design of experiments, a compromise between optimizing for discriminating between rival models and for fitting the best of them is a key point.

Once the data are collected a model has to be chosen after a model discrimination procedure, then in a second step it has to be fitted. Thus, the optimal design in this case faces two different objectives. On the one hand, it has to be good for discriminating between models. This means to organize the experiment in such a way some distances between the fitted models from the data are as large as possible to make clear the differences between them Atkinson and Fedorov (1975a), Atkinson and Fedorov (1975b), López-Fidalgo et al. (2007b), Atkinson (2008), Tommasi and López-Fidalgo (2010), Braess and Dette (2013), Tommasi et al. (2016). Appropriate distances need to be chosen according to the existing statistical tests for discriminating Cox (1962). On the other hand, the design has to be good for inferences with the chosen model, either for estimating the parameters, estimating some functions of them, or making predictions. Even for a linear model this is not trivial at all.

There are different approaches to this issue with some controversial and therefore some unclear features of them. Optimal designs from different reasonable perspectives may be rather different even for simple models. There is the need of investigating this issue providing clear directions to model selection. One of the first attempts to tackle the discrimination paradigm from an OED point of view consisted in embedding two (or more) rival models in a more general model and designing to estimate the additional parameters (Atkinson, 1972; Atkinson & Cox, 1974). This is the so-called D_s-optimal design, which makes much sense from an intuitive point of view. As a matter of fact, López-Fidalgo et al. (2008b) have proved that T- and D_s-optimality coincide only in the case that the optimal values of the parameters in the T-criterion are the nominal values for the D_s-criterion. Otherwise, the designs could be rather different. Pukelsheim and Rosenberger (1993) considered three different approaches based on compound criteria related to each rival model. This is just a compromise for estimating each of the models, but not necessarily for discriminating.

Another intuitive idea is to maximize the distance between two models by assuming that one of them is considered to be the "true" model, which is the model in the alternative hypothesis (T-optimality) (Atkinson & Fedorov, 1975a, 1975b; López-Fidalgo et al., 2007b). It turns out that this focuses on maximizing the noncentrality parameter of the likelihood ratio test statistic, which is a function of the test power. The traditional F discrimination test is a particular case for nested linear models. This criterion will be extended to the generalized linear models (GLMs) (Ponce de Leon & Atkinson, 1992) as well as to heteroscedasticity and multiple response (Ucinski & Bogacka, 2004). As a definitive extension of

T-optimality, López-Fidalgo et al. (2007b) gave a criterion based on the Kullback–Leibler distance, KL-optimality, which represents the power of the likelihood ratio test, which is also related to the Akaike Information Criterion (AIC). In particular, assuming only two rival models with pdfs

$$f_i(y, x, \theta_i), \qquad i = 1, 2,$$

and assuming f_t is the "true" model for either $t = 1$ or $t = 2$, the Kullback–Leibler distance between them is

$$\mathcal{I}(f_t, f_i, x, \theta_i) = \int f_t(y, x, \theta_t) \log \left[\frac{f_t(y, x, \theta_t)}{f_i(y, x, \theta_i)} \right] dy,$$

where $i \neq t$, y is the vector of responses, θ_i and θ_t are the parameters in the two models, and x is the vector of experimental conditions at which the response y is observed.

Then, KL-optimality is defined by the following objective function,

$$I_{i,t}(\xi) = \min_{\theta_i \in \Omega_i} \int_{\mathcal{X}} \mathcal{I}\left[f_t(y, x, \theta_t), f_i(y, x, \theta_i)\right] \xi(dx).$$

The relationship with the celebrated AIC criterion is illustrated as follows. Let $\ell_i(\theta_i)$ and $\ell_t(\theta_t)$ be the log-likelihoods of each model. It is assumed that θ_t^* is known. Then

$$\min_{\theta_i}(f_t, f_i, x, \theta_i) = E_t[L_t(\theta_t^*)] - \max_{\theta_i} E_t[L_i(\theta_i)],$$

where E_t stands for the expectation according to distribution given by f_t. The expected Akaike criterion for model i is

$$E_t[AIC_i] = 2\{m_i - E_t[L_i(\hat{\theta}_i)]\},$$

where m_i is the number of parameters of model i and $\hat{\theta}_i$ is the maximum likelihood estimator of θ_i,

$$\hat{\theta}_i = \arg\max_{\theta_i} \ell_i(\theta_i).$$

Thus, assuming the minimum can be exchanged with the expectation, then KL-optimality will minimize the AIC of model i.

López-Fidalgo et al. (2007b) proved also that T-optimality and extensions are particular cases of KL-optimality. Actually, this criterion can be used for nonnormal models or even for correlated observations (Campos-Barreiro and López-Fidalgo 2016). The criterion has been generalized in different ways for more than two rival models, essentially assuming convex combinations of the efficiencies for several models (Tommasi, 2007). Following this idea Tommasi et al. (2016) considered a max-min criterion. Compound criteria with D-optimality have been used to search for good designs also for fitting the model (Tommasi, 2009). The computational issue still needs a lot of work (Deldossi et al., 2016).

Recently, Lanteri et al. (2023) proved some properties relating KL-optimality and D_s-optimality with the maximization of the noncentrality parameter of the asymptotic chi-squared distribution of a likelihood-based test for discriminating heteroscedasticity in a nonlinear Gaussian regression model. Specifically, when the variance function depends just on one parameter, the two criteria coincide asymptotically and in particular, the D_1-criterion is proportional to the noncentrality parameter. Differently, if the variance function depends on a vector of parameters, then the KL-optimum design converges to the design that maximizes the noncentrality parameter.

Summarizing all this, model selection is an important topic in contemporary statistics and the OED perspective can provide a significant improvement to this problem. Finding a joint solution to the problem of identifying the maximum information, both to discriminate between rival models and to better fit them, remains a challenging issue.

5.5.1 Bayesian Paradigm

Most of the optimality criteria focus on the inverse of the information matrix. If the model is nonlinear, the FIM depends on the model parameters. KL-optimality, and thus T-optimality, does not focus on this matrix but directly on the probability measure, that is, the design. However, even for linear models, nominal values of the parameters of the "true" model are needed. One way to address this issue is the use of the Bayesian paradigm assuming a prior distribution on the parameters and a joint utility function that includes both objectives at the same time, estimating the model parameters and finding the optimal design for it. Tommasi and López-Fidalgo (2010) introduced the Bayesian approach to discriminate between two rival models avoiding the annoying "true model" assumption.

Utility functions focused on discrimination should be considered. This is very much related again to finding different measures of divergence. Some, but not all, of the classic optimization criteria have a Bayesian version based on utility. Combining utility functions can help describe several simultaneous goals. Furthermore, Tommasi et al. (2016) considered a maximin criterion for more than two rival models and gave a relationship with a Bayesian criterion assuming a prior distribution of the weights of each model. This particular point can be explored using mathematical programming techniques applied here. This would be very useful for computational purposes. The maximin criteria are not easy to handle due to the lack of differentiability. The GET is still applicable, but an annoying auxiliary probability measure must be found.

Thus, the Bayesian paradigm brings a convincing way of dealing with the unknown parameters, better justified criteria that do not rely on the artificial assumption of a "true" model and a nice way of dealing with more than two rival models.

5.5.2 Correlated Observations

The field of Big Data is a world of correlations, which must be considered from different perspectives. Unlike other discrimination criteria, KL-optimality is still valid in this situation. Campos-Barreiro and López-Fidalgo (2016) showed that a standard generalization of T-optimality can be made to correlated observations just when the covariance matrix of the observations is assumed to be completely known. Models with a partially unknown covariance structure have been extensively studied. Most of this work has been done for D-optimality. The approximation of the covariance matrix by the inverse of the FIM holds in this situation under some assumptions. If these conditions are not met, simulations with the designs obtained in the last steps of the algorithm to check the monotonicity between the determinants of the FIM and the covariance matrix would be enough. KL-optimality is not based on the FIM. Therefore, there is no problem with the mentioned approximation.

Much work can be done in the area of optimal designs for discrimination in the presence of correlated observations. In particular, the usual time series models require a discrimination process to select the best model, for example, the best values of p, d, and q in an ARIMA(p, d, q) model. This is an area where things are not so simple from an experimental design point of view. Amo-Salas et al. (2015) considered a fairly simple time series model where the implicit covariance structure is computed from the model. This can be done analytically on very simple models, but it needs some new results to be able to find a suitable criterion for both discriminating and estimating the models.

5.5.3 Computing Optimal Designs

While iterative procedures are very much needed for OED in general, they are specially needed for finding optimal information for discriminating between models. For KL-optimality some classical algorithms have been adapted, but much more work has to be done here. López-Fidalgo et al. (2007b) provided a general algorithm based on the directional derivative,

(i) For a given design ξ_s let

$$\theta_{i,s} = \arg\min_{\theta_i \in \Omega_i} \int \mathcal{I}(f_t, f_i, x, \theta_i)\xi_s(dx)$$

$$x_s = \arg\max_{x \in \chi} \mathcal{I}(f_t, f_i, x, \theta_{i,s}).$$

(ii) For a chosen α_s with $0 \leq \alpha_s \leq 1$ let

$$\xi_{s+1} = (1 - \alpha_s)\xi_s + \alpha_s \xi_{x_s},$$

where ξ_{x_s} is a design with measure concentrated at the single point x_s.
For convergence typical conditions for the sequences $\{\alpha_s\}$ are

$$\lim_{s \to \infty} \alpha_s = 0, \quad \sum_{s=0}^{\infty} \alpha_s = \infty, \quad \sum_{s=0}^{\infty} \alpha_s^2 < \infty.$$

This algorithm becomes slow after a while and needs to be combined with a finer algorithm in the last part of the procedure. Tommasi et al. (2016) provided another algorithm, this time for a max-min criterion considering more than two rival models. Convenient algorithms need to be adapted to this criterion and then their performance need to be evaluated.

5.6 Meta-heuristic Algorithm

In Chap. 2.7 the Wynn–Fedorov algorithm (Wynn, 1970) and a multiplicative algorithm (see also Torsney, 1983; Mandal & Torsney, 2000; Martin-Martin et al., 2007; Harman, 2014) were introduced. Both are efficient for reasonable dimensions, but they become inefficient when the number of parameters and variables increases (Wu & Wynn, 1978). Fedorov (1989) considered an algorithm quite interesting at this respect. Harman and Lacko (2010) developed decompositional algorithms for uniform sampling. Filova et al. (2012), Duarte and Wong (2014) adapted semidefinite programming to the computation of optimal designs. Yang et al. (2013) considered a very simple but very efficient algorithm. The design points are computed by using the directional derivative based on the equivalence theorem. Then, at each step, the best weights for those points are computed using traditional algorithms, such as Newton–Rapson. Sagnol and Harman (2015) used mixed integer second-order cone programming for computing exact D-optimal designs. Harman et al. (2016), Harman and Benkova (2017) provided algorithms under multiple resource constraints. Harman et al. (2020) developed a randomized exchange algorithm for computing optimal approximate designs. It is quite interesting the approach of Rosa and Harman (2022) for computing minimum-volume enclosing ellipsoids for large datasets. Chapter 9 of the monograph by Pronzato and Pázman (2013) provided a good and extensive review of numerical algorithms.

Optimal experimental design computation is actually an area that needs much exploration. In recent years this is starting to be an important area of interest (e.g., Duarte & Wong, 2014; García-Ródenas et al., 2020; Harman & Rosa, 2020). The meta-heuristic algorithms, many of them nature-inspired, are rather fast, although convergence is not guaranteed. Some intensive research in this area can be seen, for instance, in Wong and Zhou (2019), Stokes et al. (2020), Duarte et al. (2020), Liu et al. (2021), Yu et al. (2023), Wong and Zhou (2023), Liu et al. (2022), Chen et al. (2022). Vazquez et al. (2023) used mixed-integer programming and heuristic algorithms for computing optimal screening designs. Additionally, some parameters have to be tuned without general directions for it. In the era of machine learning tuning the initial parameters of an algorithm is a challenge. These parameters control the trade-off between exploration (of the whole domain) and exploitation (capability of reaching the top of the local optima). Here it happens that the theory of optimal experimental design can help to check the most informative values of the initial parameters to tune them optimally.

An efficient algorithm is a compromise between precision of the solution and speediness. Usually, for exact algorithms more weight is put in precision than in computation time. It is worth to mention that these type of heuristic algorithms do not pay so much attention to the precision. The typical way of acting is fixing a computation time, that is, a number of iterations, and then run the algorithm and check the solution. It is quite usual to run the algorithm several times, even with different values of the parameters of the algorithm, and then take the best solution. This is because the behavior, and so the convergence, of the algorithm is not well-known and it is better to try several times than running the algorithm until some stopping rule is fulfilled. This last chance may take forever if we were not lucky with the initial solutions or the tuning parameters.

We are considering a couple of meta-heuristic algorithms adapted to the computation of optimal experimental designs to show the potential of these population algorithms.

5.6.1 *Particle Swarm Optimization (PSO)*

The main idea of this algorithm is the behavior of a group of organized living beings such as a group of birds migrating in that particular crib shape. Thus, the algorithm starts with a population of birds (designs in our case) and they move all together taking advantage of the individual expertise, on the one hand, and the group expertise, on the other hand. Some inertia are usually considered as well. Thus, a particular bird moves as a resultant of three vectors. One vector is defined by the inertia, a second one corresponds to its best experience along the way, and the other

Table 5.5 Values of the criterion function evaluated at each of the designs computed until step s

Step	Design	1	...	N	Optimal
0		$\Phi_1^{(0)}$	...	$\Phi_N^{(0)}$	$\Phi^{(0)\star}$
1		$\Phi_1^{(1)}$	...	$\Phi_N^{(1)}$	$\Phi^{(1)\star}$
...	...	...	...	...	
s		$\Phi_1^{(s)}$	...	$\Phi_N^{(s)}$	$\Phi^{(s)\star}$
	Optimal	$\Phi_1^{(s)\star}$	...	$\Phi_N^{(s)\star}$	

vector is determined by the best experience of the group. The weights of each of the last two vectors are the product of a fixed parameter for the whole algorithm and a random value computed at each step. This is a version of the algorithm adapted to optimal experimental design,

1. Let $\xi_1^{(0)}, \ldots, \xi_N^{(0)}$ be the initial population of designs, considered as the initial positions of the birds.
2. After s steps the new population of designs is formed by $\xi_1^{(s)}, \ldots, \xi_N^{(s)}$. At this point Table 5.5 collects the criterion function evaluated at each design, where $\Phi_j^{(s)\star} = \min\{\Phi_j^{(0)}, \Phi_j^{(1)}, \ldots, \Phi_j^{(s)}\}$ is the optimal value of the trajectory of design (bird) $j = 1, \ldots, N$. This design will be called $\xi_j^{(s)\star}$. The value $\Phi^{(s)\star} = \min\{\Phi_1^{(s)\star}, \Phi_2^{(s)\star} \ldots, \Phi_N^{(s)\star}\}$ is the optimal in the whole table until step s. It will be called $\xi^{(s)\star}$.
3. The new designs at step $s+1$ are then

$$\xi_j^{(s+1)} = \xi_j^{(s)} + v_j^{(s+1)},$$

   where the velocity is computed as

$$v_j^{(s+1)} = wv_j^{(s+1)} + \alpha \bullet [R_1 \bullet (\xi_j^{(s)\star} - \xi_j^{(s)})] + \beta \bullet [R_2 \bullet (\xi^{(s)\star} - \xi_j^{(s)})]$$

4. The process is repeated until

$$\frac{\Phi^{(s)\star} - \Phi^{(s+1)\star}}{\Phi^{(s)\star}} \leq \delta \text{ (e.g., 0.01)}.$$

   For approximate designs this can also be stated in terms of efficiencies according to the bounds of different criteria given in Sect. 2.6.2.

The tuning parameters and the operators $+$ and $\bullet$ need some explanation:

Population size (N). It needs to be big enough, but not too big, taking into account the computational cost increases considerably with it.

Inertia parameter (w). It should be between zero and one.

α, β are called cognitive and social coefficients, respectively. They are two-dimensional vectors with typical components between 1 and 3, fixed from the beginning. They are in charge of giving the adequate weight to the points and the probabilities of the design for each of the vectors defining the movement. They are two-dimensional since using different numbers for the points and for the probabilities is quite advisable.

R_1, R_2 are two-dimensional vectors with random components from the uniform distribution on (0, 1) generated at each step of the algorithm.

Operators $+, -$ mean here summing or subtracting the support points of the designs and all the weights, but the last one, which will be computed at the end of all operations subtracting to 1 the sum of the weights, but the last one.

Operator $\bullet$ means multiplying the first component of the two-dimensional vector by the support points of the designs. Then the second component multiplies all the weights, but the last one, which will be computed in such a way the sum of the final weights is 1.

Summarizing this more explicitly,

$$\begin{Bmatrix} a \\ b \end{Bmatrix} \bullet \begin{Bmatrix} x_1 & \cdots & x_k \\ p_1 & \cdots & p_k \end{Bmatrix} + \begin{Bmatrix} z_1 & \cdots & z_k \\ q_1 & \cdots & q_k \end{Bmatrix} =$$

$$\begin{Bmatrix} ax_1 + z_1 & \cdots & ax_{k-1} + z_{k-1} & ax_k + z_k \\ bp_1 + q_1 & \cdots & bp_{k-1} + q_{k-1} & w \end{Bmatrix},$$

where $w = 1 - (bp_1 + q_1) - \cdots - (bp_{k-1} + q_{k-1})$.

To keep the points in the design space and the weights coherent during the algorithm, the value of the criterion function of a candidate not satisfying the conditions to be within these spaces will be strongly penalized to be discarded by the algorithm.

5.6.2 Genetic Algorithm

This algorithm emulates the process of natural genetic selection in three different steps: reproduction, mutation, and elitist selection. It is introduced here for computing Φ-optimal approximate designs in a very simple way (see, e.g., Broudiscou et al., 1996 for a simple and clear introduction). An approximate experimental design (*chromosome*) for a model with p variables is of the form

$$\xi = \begin{Bmatrix} (x_{11}, \ldots, x_{1p}) & \cdots & (x_{k1}, \ldots, x_{kp}) \\ p_1 & \cdots & p_k \end{Bmatrix},$$

where $(x_{11}, \ldots, x_{1p}) \in \chi \subset \mathbb{R}^p$. Each chromosome has to be divided in *genes*. In this case, the $kp + k$ genes can be considered

$$x_{11} \ldots x_{1p} p_1 \cdots x_{k1} \ldots x_{kp} p_k.$$

Sometimes a binary codification of each number (gene) is used. Thus, previous chromosome may have a form like this

$$0111010001011000111110100010100011110,$$

where the limits of each gene are known.

The starting step of the algorithm consist in generating randomly a population of N chromosomes, for example, $N = 50$.

Reproduction: A number of random pairs are formed, for example, $N/2$ pairs. For each pair,

$$\xi = x_{11} \ldots x_{1p} p_1 \cdots x_{k1} \ldots x_{kp} p_k,$$
$$\xi' = x'_{11} \ldots x'_{1p} p'_1 \cdots x'_{k1} \ldots x'_{kp} p'_k,$$

each gene is selected with probability P_c, typically in the interval $[0.7, 1)$. Those selected in the first chromosome are exchanged with the corresponding ones of the second chromosome. The new chromosome is an *offspring*. Usually, one or two are generated from each pair.

Mutation: Each gene of an offspring is selected or not with probability P_m, typically in the interval $[0.001, 0.05]$. Those selected are substituted by one generated randomly in the corresponding space.

Elitist selection: The original parent population and the offspring population are joined. Then the worse according to the optimality criterion are discarded. Typically, $N/2$ could be discarded so the size of the population is still N.

The process goes on until some number of steps or until a stopping rule is satisfied for the best chromosome obtained. In all cases the weights of the designs have to be normalized to be between zero and one and to sum up to one.

The tuning parameters are:

N, which needs to be big enough, but not too big, taking into account computational cost increases considerably with it. A trade-off between exploitation and exploration has to be taken into account.

k, which can be determined according to the expected number of points of the optimal design. There is always the limit stabilized by Caratheodory's theorem.

offspring size, which needs to be tuned again for optimal speed and convergence.

Remark 5.4 It is worthwhile to mention that there is not a canonical version of the algorithm. What is important is the idea of the procedure and the phases in it. For instance, instead of exchanging or mutating whole genes, just some parts can be exchanged, stabilizing one or several cut-offs along the chromosome. Sometimes there is an intermediate division of the chromosome in *bitfields*, which will be divided again in *genes*.

Example 5.3 The Michaelis Menten Model is revisited here,

$$y = \frac{Vx}{x+K} + \varepsilon,\ x \in [0, bK].$$

with the usual conditions of normality, independence, and homoscedasticity. López Fidalgo and Wong (2002) gave the D-optimal design,

$$\xi_D^\star = \left\{ \begin{matrix} \frac{b}{2+b}K & bK \\ 1/2 & 1/2 \end{matrix} \right\}.$$

Thus, algorithms are not needed, but we are using this simple example of a nonlineal model to show how the algorithms explained so far work. First, the nonlinear model is linearized around the nominal values of the parameters $(V_0, K_0) = (1, 1)$,

$$y = V\frac{x}{x+1} - K\frac{x}{(x+1)^2} + \varepsilon,\ \chi = [0, 5].$$

The FIM for a design ξ is then

$$M(\xi) = \sum_{x\in[0,5]} \xi(x) \begin{pmatrix} \frac{x^2}{(x+1)^2} & \frac{-x^2}{(x+1)^3} \\ \frac{-x^2}{(x+1)^3} & \frac{x^2}{(x+1)^4} \end{pmatrix}$$

We know the D-optimal design is in this case

$$\xi_D^\star = \left\{ \begin{matrix} 0.71 & 5 \\ 1/2 & 1/2 \end{matrix} \right\}.$$

Wynn–Fedorov Algorithm (Sect. 2.7.1)

The first-order algorithm is developed here step by step. Let an initial design be

$$\xi_0 = \left\{ \begin{matrix} 1 & 4 \\ 1/2 & 1/2 \end{matrix} \right\}.$$

Its information matrix is

$$M(\xi_0) = \begin{pmatrix} 0.45 & -0.13 \\ -0.13 & 0.044 \end{pmatrix},$$

and the inverse

$$M^{-1}(\xi_0) = \begin{pmatrix} 12.2 & 35.1 \\ 35.1 & 123.6 \end{pmatrix}.$$

The maximum of the sensitivity function $d(x, \xi_0) = x^2[4721 + x(-3298 + 881x)]/72(x+1)^4$ is reached at $x_0 = 0.63$ and a new design constructed

$$\xi_1 = 1/2\xi_0 + 1/2\xi_{x_0} = \begin{Bmatrix} 0.63 & 1 & 4 \\ 1/2 & 1/4 & 1/4 \end{Bmatrix}.$$

Repeating the process once again, $x_1 = 5$ and

$$\xi_2 = 2/3\xi_1 + 1/3\xi_{x_1} = \begin{Bmatrix} 0.63 & 1 & 4 & 5 \\ 1/3 & 1/6 & 1/6 & 1/3 \end{Bmatrix}.$$

Now $x_2 = 0.69$ and the Atwood bound of the efficiency can be computed as 0.97, giving a good design approximating the D-optimal. The algorithm is good at the beginning, but it becomes quite slow to get a high efficiency.

Multiplicative Algorithm (Sect. 2.7.2)

The design space is discretized as $\chi = \{0, 0.1, 0.2, \ldots, 4.8, 4.9, 5\}$. Actually, one decimal is quite enough for this model. Consider an initial design including all the points with positive weights (all equal),

$$\xi_0 = \begin{Bmatrix} 0 & 0.1 & \cdots & 5 \\ 1/51 & 1/51 & \cdots & 1/51 \end{Bmatrix}.$$

The inverse of the FIM is then

$$M^{-1}(\xi_0) = \begin{pmatrix} 15.89 & 50.57 \\ 50.57 & 187.26 \end{pmatrix},$$

and the sensitivity function $d(x, \xi_0) = x^2[102.0 + x(-64.4 + 15.9x)]/(x+1)^4$. Then the new weights are computed as follows:

$$\xi_1(0) = \xi_0(0)\frac{d(0, \xi_0)}{2} = 0,\ \xi_1(0.1) = \xi_0(0.1)\frac{d(0.1, \xi_0)}{2} = 0.063,$$
$$\ldots \xi_1(0.7) = \xi_0(0.7)\frac{d(0.7, \xi_0)}{2} = 0.035, \ldots$$

That is,

$$\xi_1 = \begin{Bmatrix} 0 & 0.1 & \cdots & 0.7 & \cdots & 5 \\ 0 & 0.0063 & \cdots & 0.035 & \cdots & 0.029 \end{Bmatrix}$$

with a bound of the efficiency of 0.55. Repeating the process we obtain

$$\xi_2 = \begin{Bmatrix} 0 & 0.1 & \cdots & 0.7 & \cdots & 5 \\ 0 & 0.0015 & \cdots & 0.048 & \cdots & 0.039 \end{Bmatrix}$$

with a bound of the efficiency of 0.74.

To get a bound greater than 0.99, we need up to 50 steps,

$$\xi_{50} = \begin{Bmatrix} 0 & 0.1 & \cdots & 0.7 & \cdots & 5 \\ 0 & 6 \times 10^{-41} & \cdots & 0.22 & \cdots & 0.33 \end{Bmatrix}.$$

Again, this algorithm is good at the beginning, but it becomes quite slow to get a high efficiency. The meta-heuristic algorithms become much faster, but they depend much on the initial parameters to be tuned.

PSO

For illustration a population with ten designs is chosen for the algorithm. Table 5.6 shows the starting population. Thus, the global leader is the third one while the leader for each trajectory at this first step is the same starting design $\xi_j^{(0)\star} = \xi_j^{(0)}$, $j = 1, \ldots, 10$. Let us assume the generated numbers from the uniform distribution are $R_1^T = (0.4, 0.8)$, $R_2^T = (0.7, 0.1)$ fixing $w = 0.5, \alpha = (1, 1)^T$ and $\beta = (1, 1)^T$. Thus,

$$\xi_j^{(1)} = \xi_j^{(0)} + [(0.4, 0.8)^T \bullet (\xi_j^{(0)\star} - \xi_j^{(0)})] + [(0.7, 0.1)^T \bullet (\xi^{(0)\star} - \xi_j^{(0)})].$$

After 50 iterations the final population reduces to the same design at points 0.708 and 5 with weights 0.5003 and 0.4997, which is very near the D-optimal design. Since the D-optimal design is known, the exact efficiency of this design can be computed, which is 0.999989. This algorithm has been run a few times, no more than ten times, until this good result was obtained. Some results were very bad. The algorithm is very fast.

In this example when a support point became negative or greater than 5, it was fixed to 0 or 5, respectively. If a weight was not between 0 and 1, then the previous weights were considered again. Many different tricks can be considered in each specific case to speed up the convergence.

Table 5.6 Initial population for the PSO algorithm with the objective values

Points	0.392	4.137	0.067	0.309	4.705	0.940	3.343	1.058	0.688	2.401
Weights	0.133	0.867	0.275	0.725	0.408	0.592	0.458	0.542	0.600	0.340
Determinant	0.00163		0.000		0.00447		0.00254		0.00177	
Points	0.402	3.395	4.963	4.051	2.207	4.904	0.00613	4.357	0.654	2.237
Weights	0.640	0.360	0.773	0.227	0.815	0.185	0.892	0.108	0.786	0.214
Determinant	0.00267		0.0000717		0.00100		0.000		0.00110	

Genetic Algorithm

In this simple example with two parameters, just two-point designs will be considered for illustrating the algorithm. Three genes are considered for each design, the two points jointly with its weight. No binary codification is used at all. All this simplifies the procedure very much. It is just to make it simple for illustration. A starting population of $N = 50$, two-point designs are randomly generated.

Reproduction: $N/2 = 25$ pairs were randomly generated. For each pair,

$$\xi = \begin{Bmatrix} x_1 & x_2 \\ p_1 & 1 - p_1 \end{Bmatrix}, \quad \xi' = \begin{Bmatrix} x_1' & x_2' \\ p_1' & 1 - p_1' \end{Bmatrix},$$

gene 1 and gene 2 were, respectively, selected or not with probability $P_c = 0.7$. Those selected in the first chromosome are exchanged with the corresponding ones of the second chromosome. The new chromosome is an *offspring*. In this simple case there are six possibilities for the offspring,

$$\xi, \quad \xi', \quad \begin{Bmatrix} x_1' & x_2 \\ p_1' & 1 - p_1' \end{Bmatrix}, \quad \begin{Bmatrix} x_1 & x_2' \\ p_1' & 1 - p_1' \end{Bmatrix}, \quad \begin{Bmatrix} x_1' & x_2 \\ p_1 & 1 - p_1 \end{Bmatrix} \text{ or } \begin{Bmatrix} x_1 & x_2' \\ p_1 & 1 - p_1 \end{Bmatrix}.$$

Mutation: Each gene of an offspring is selected or not with probability $P_m = 0.05$. Those selected are substituted by one generated randomly in $[0, 5]$ for the points and $[0, 1]$ for the weight.

Elitist selection: The original parent population and the offspring population were joined. Then the worse 25, according to the optimality criterion, were discarded.

The whole process was iterated 50 times and the following design was obtained with an efficiency of 0.996,

$$\begin{Bmatrix} 0.726892 & 4.9603 \\ 0.494146 & 0.505854 \end{Bmatrix}.$$

Exercise 5.1 Compute a KL-optimal design for simple linear regression for $\chi = [-1, 1]$ assuming independent errors with Normality in one model and the t-student distribution with three degrees of freedom in the rival model, that is,

$$\varepsilon \sim \mathcal{N}(0, \sigma^2) \text{ versus } \varepsilon \sim \mathrm{t}_3$$

The nominal values to be considered are $\theta_0 = \theta_1 = 1$ and the variance is common in both cases and known ($\sigma = 3$). Assume the "true" model is the Normal distribution.

Solution (Hints:) The pdfs for the two distributions of the observations are, respectively,

$$h_1(y, \theta_0, \theta_1) = \frac{1}{\sqrt{6\pi}} e^{-\frac{1}{6}(y-\theta_0-\theta_1 x)^2},$$

$$h_2(y, \theta_0, \theta_1) = \frac{1}{\sqrt{3\pi}\Gamma(3/2)} \left[1 + \frac{(y-\theta_0-\theta_1 x)^2}{3}\right]^{-2}.$$

Exercise 5.2 Make a code in the computer language of your choice for implementing the algorithms given in this chapter for computing D-optimal designs for the quadratic model.

Chapter 6
Real Case Examples

6.1 Introduction

In this chapter a few illustrative examples for nonstandard situations are provided. An example for correlated observations related to retention of radiation in the human body shows the impact of this topic. Designs for modeling through a mixture of distributions have not been very much considered in the literature, although they appear to be very useful to model a variety of real situations. The problem of identifiability needs here a deep consideration. Then, computing the FIM, and so optimal designs, becomes a very challenging goal. This is shown as an emerging topic for future research. OED makes sense whenever a variable can be controlled by an experimenter, in a broader sense. It is usual to assume in this case that all the explanatory variables are under control, frequently just one. But in real scenarios there are mixture of variables under control jointly with uncontrolled variables, whose values come randomly. This is a nonstandard situation at all considered here.

In the real world some potential censoring emerges frequently. For instance, when the time of an exercise or any other experiment is designed, the exercise may be stopped before reaching the time targeted in the optimal design. This has to be taken into account in advance to compute "optimal expected designs." This is censoring in the explanatory variable under control, but the typical censoring in survival models introduces an important degree of complexity when a design is being optimized before knowing which experimental units are going to be censored.

In previous chapters everything has been explained in such a way that the reader should be able to reproduce the techniques introduced there in detail. This has been the aim of the book, teaching the "knowhow" of OED. This last chapter shows motivating real applications of the theory of OED. Most of them were researched by the author and they are not so simple to be explained here in detail. That would take too much space and this is not the purpose of the book. Most of them need new methodology; they are actually the material of several papers. This chapter tries to be just an eyeview of real applications after giving the general theory. The examples

J. López-Fidalgo, *Optimal Experimental Design*, Lecture Notes in Statistics 226,
https://doi.org/10.1007/978-3-031-35918-7_6

prove how this topic relates the researcher with different areas of statistics as well as different sciences and areas. Thus, this chapter has to be read with a different disposition trying to understand the general ideas. For details he or she can go to the cited papers.

6.2 Mixture of Distributions: Engine Emissions

This problem comes from the group of machines and engines of the Engineering School of Castilla-La Mancha in Ciudad Real, Spain. Experiments with a combustion engine are realized in different conditions and emissions of several types of particles are measured. The objective is to reduce the pollution in the atmosphere caused by cars. The response variable is the diameter of the particles, knowing there are several types of particles, which can be distinguished by the size. There is interest in estimating the proportion of particles of each kind since some types of particles are more toxic than others. On the other hand, there may be interest also in estimating the parameters of each population. Thus, a mixture of distributions model has to be considered. A first problem is that computing MLEs is rather difficult in this case with the additional issue of identifiability. The Expectation-Maximization (EM) algorithm for missing data is used in this context for approximating the MLEs. Figure 6.1 shows some examples of different experiments. The mixture of two normal distributions is quite clear showing two different types of particles distinguished by their size. Figure 6.2 shows different possible theoretical cases of mixture of normal distributions.

In a general framework for a mixture of two populations, the distribution of the response, y, at given values of covariates, x, is given by a pdf

$$f_Y(y|x,\theta) = (1-p) f_0(y|x,\theta) + p f_1(y|x,\theta),$$

where $f_0(y|x,\theta)$ and $f_1(y|x,\theta)$ are the pdfs of the two distributions with means $\mu_0 = \alpha_0 + \beta_0 x$, $\mu_1 = \alpha_1 + \beta_1 x$ and variances σ_0, σ_1. If n_j independent experiments are performed for each value x_j, $n = \sum_{j=1}^k n_j$, then some observations y_{ij}, $i = 1, \ldots, n_j$, $j = 1, \ldots, k$ are recorded. Then the following probabilities

$$u_{ij} = P(Z=1|Y=y_{ij}) = \frac{p f_1(y_{ij}|x_j,\theta)}{(1-p) f_0(y_{ij}|x_j,\theta) + p f_1(y_{ij}|x_j,\theta)},$$

can be computed after giving some values to the parameters. The EM algorithm consists in recalculating u_{ij}, $i = 1, \ldots, n_j$, $j = 1, \ldots, k$ at each step updating the values of the parameters. For instance, the recurrent estimate of p is

$$\widehat{p} = \frac{1}{\sum_{j=1}^k n_j} \sum_{j=1}^k \sum_{i=1}^{n_j} u_{ij}.$$

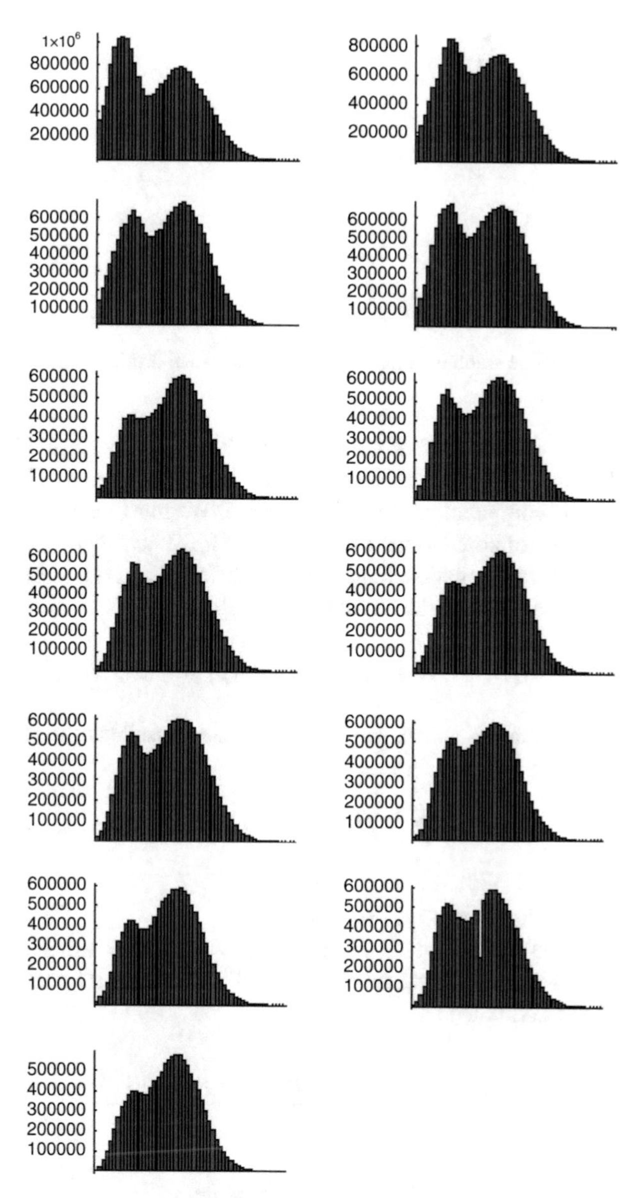

Fig. 6.1 Histograms of sizes of 13 big samples of contaminating particles with real data

There is an important problem here to obtain a closed form of the FIM since the mixture of two distributions of the exponential family is not usually within this family. This means the FIM or the covariance matrix of the estimators has to be approximated, for example,

- Using simulations:

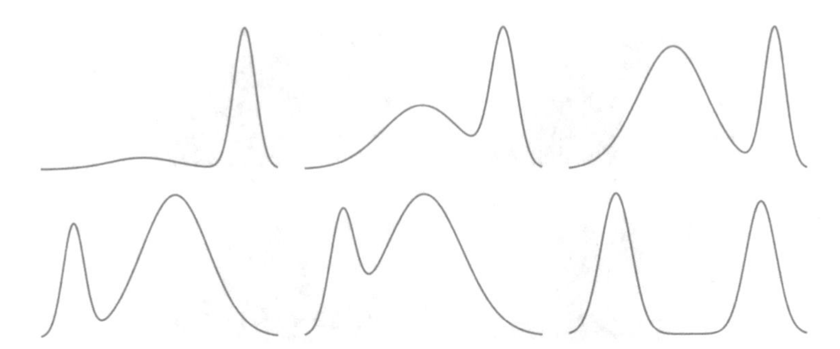

Fig. 6.2 Different possible theoretical cases of mixture of normal distributions

- Through the empirical covariance matrix. This is rather effective since no approximation of this matrix through the FIM is considered. The problem is that it can be computationally nonaffordable. We must take into account that a large number of simulations has to be done for "each" design candidate.
- Simulating the information matrix at the different values of the discretized design space is much cheaper computationally,

$$I(x_1, \theta), \ \ldots, \ I(x_k, \theta), \ \theta^T = (p, \ \alpha_0, \ \beta_0, \ \alpha_1, \ \beta_1).$$

Then the information matrix can be built for any possible design,

$$M(\xi) = \sum_{j=1}^{k} \xi_j I(x_j, \theta), \ \xi_j \geq 0, \ \sum_{i=1}^{k} \xi_j = 1,$$

and integrated in an iterative procedure.
In particular, at each point x_j, N responses $y_{j1}, \ldots, y_{jN}$ are simulated using the nominal values of the parameters, say $\theta^{(0)}$. Then the one-point information matrix is approximated as

$$I(x_j, \theta^{(0)}) \approx \sum_{r=1}^{N} \frac{\partial^2 \log h(y_{jr}|x_j, \theta^{(0)})}{\partial \theta}.$$

- Directly using Taylor approximations, for example,
  - approximating $f_Y(y|x, \theta)$ or
  - approximating the terms of the FIM by $\frac{\partial \eta(x,\theta)}{\partial \theta} \frac{\partial \eta(x,\theta)}{\partial \theta^T}$.

Example with a Mixture of Two Normal Distributions

Here we choose simulating for approximating the FIM. $N = 10,000$ simulations are going to be performed at each of the 11 points $\{0, 0.1, 0.2, \ldots, 1\}$ of the discretized design space $[0, 1]$. Different D-optimal designs,

$$\left\{ \begin{matrix} 0 & 1 \\ p_0 & 1 - p_0 \end{matrix} \right\},$$

are shown in Table 6.1 for several nominal values of the parameters.

For the computations just two-point designs were considered. Therefore, the equivalence theorem needed to be checked with the best two-point design. Figure 6.3 shows for one example that the maximum of the sensitivity function for D-optimality, $m - \text{tr}[M(\xi_x)M(\xi)]$, is over 0 for $m = 7$ parameters to be estimated.

Table 6.1 D-optimal design: p_0 is the weight of the right extreme value 1

Nominal values							D-optimal
p	α_0	α_1	β_0	β_1	σ_0^2	σ_1^2	p_0
0.2	1	2	3	3	1	1	0.405
0.6	1	2	3	3	1	1	0.406
0.6	1	2	3	3	0.5	1	0.404
0.15	1	2	3	3	0.5	1	0.404
0.3	1	2	3	3	0.5	0.3	0.414
0.5	1	2	3	3	1	0.2	0.419
0.8	1	2	3	3	1	0.1	0.442

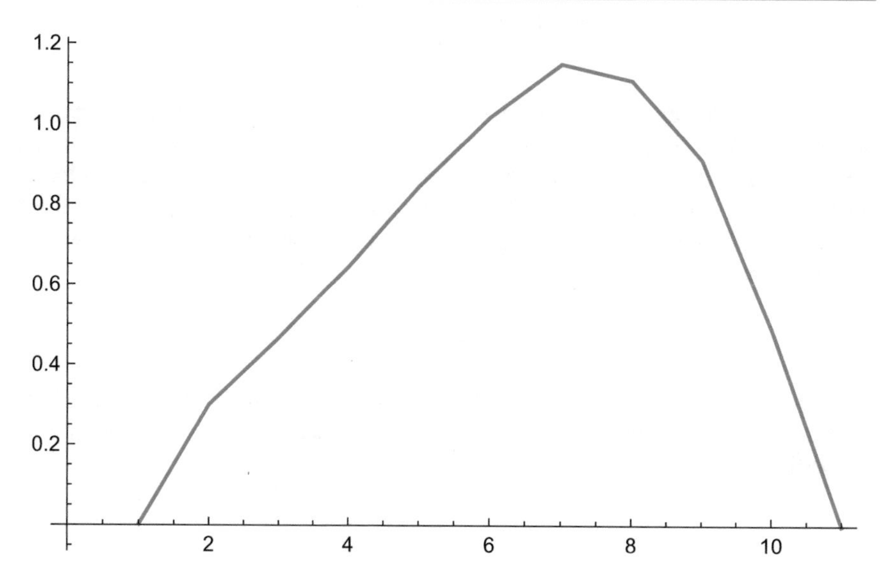

Fig. 6.3 Sensitivity function for D-optimality

6.3 Correlated Observations and Spatial Models: Radiation Retention in the Human Body

An important part of our research in optimal experimental design has been in collaboration with Guillermo Sánchez and some other people of the factory ENUSA INDUSTRIAS AVANZADAS, S.A. (Salamanca, Spain). Actually, we have a number of publications based on this situation, where details may be checked (López-Fidalgo et al., 2005; López-Fidalgo & Sanchez, 2005; López-Fidalgo & Villarroel, 2007; Sánchez, 2007; Sánchez & Rodríguez-Díaz, 2007). This factory produces the final product for nuclear plants after a final process of the enriched uranium received. Typically, the radiation retention in the human body is modeled by a compartmental model, where the parts of the body, including the blood, are compartments (around 15–20). This takes to a graph with a number of nodes (compartments) and arrows showing the transference of the radiation between compartments with a particular transfer rate. These models are well-studied and they have known coefficients for different substances given in different documents of the International Commission on Radiological Protection (ICRP).

In a possible accidental radioactive leak in a uranium factory, a worker may receive an initial intake, I, of particles of size s. The protocol in a case like this asks for a first immediate bioassay, say at time t_1. After some time another bioassay has to be made to estimate the value of the unknown initial intake, I. The graph of compartmental models provides a large system of linear differential equations. The solutions provide a model of the radiation elimination (retention) from the human body. This solution is a sum of a number of exponentials, typically

$$q(t, s) = I \sum_j \gamma_j e^{-\alpha s - \beta t},$$

where all the coefficients are assumed known here but I that should be estimated. We have used the theory of optimal experimental design for optimizing the second time, t_2. Since two or more observations are measured in the subject, the correlation between them has to be taken into account through a covariance structure, for example, a triangular one depending just on the time elapsed between observations but not on the particle size,

$$\text{cov}(y_{(t,s)}, y_{(t',s')}) = \sigma^2(1 - |t - t'|/\theta_2).$$

Table 6.2 shows some results for this model and correlation structure. It is interesting to see that there is a jump when the correlation increases depending on the particle size.

Table 6.2 Optimal second point for the triangular correlation for $t_1 = 0.5$

$s \setminus \theta_2$	1	5	10	50
2	90.14	92.43	90.09	1.09
5	69.56	70.14	1.13	1.12
6	63.55	1.16	1.10	1.13
10	58.06	1.16	1.11	1.14

6.4 Marginally Restricted Designs: Uranium Densification

Coming back to the uranium factory a different problem is considered now. They produce uranium rods consisting in an ensemble of tubes containing pellets made with uranium. The pellets need a specific density and porosity since pores are to retain fission gases during the heating in the reactor of the nuclear plant. To obtain appropriate pores some additives are merged with the uranium dust. Then the mass is heated in a furnace during a specified time. During this process the additives are burned off forming pores. To optimize the porosity a two-degree polynomial is fitted using as explanatory variables the "Initial density," s, which is not under the control of the practitioner; the "percentage of additive U_3O_8," t, which can be controlled; and the "final density," y, that is the result (response) of the experiment,

$$y = \gamma_0 + \gamma_1 s + \gamma_2 t + \gamma_{12} st + \gamma_{11} s^2 + \gamma_{22} t^2 + \varepsilon.$$

The initial density s goes from 94.9% to 96.7% in this particular sample while the percentage of additive has to be chosen for each density between 0% and 20%. A covariance structure was convenient taking into account the unique process. The following structure was appropriate,

$$\text{cov}(y, y') = \sigma^2 exp\big[(1/\theta_2 - 1)|s - s'|^{\theta_2} + |t - t'|^{\theta_2}\big],\ 0 < \theta_2 < 1.$$

This function has just two parameters, what makes it quite affordable, both from the estimation and the optimal experimental points of view. Using historical data an estimated value $\hat{\theta}_2 = 0.93$ was obtained with the usual two-step algorithm,

1. An initial value of the covariance parameters is guessed and then the parameters of the mean are estimated.
2. With the estimated parameters of the means, the covariance parameters are now estimated.
3. The process is repeated until some stopping rule based on the variation of the estimation of the parameters is met.

This value provides the following covariance structure:

$$\text{cov}(y, y') = \sigma^2 exp\big[0.075|s - s'|^{0.93} + |t - t'|^{0.93}\big],$$

which means there is a low impact of the initial density in correlation, while the percentage of additive induces some correlation.

A sample of 392 units were used for the experiment. The "Initial density" of each of them is measured before. Thus, the marginal distribution of variable s is completely known, say $\tilde{\xi}_1$. The units have to be heated in the furnace to get the pellets. Then we need to find an optimal conditional design given each of these values, say $\xi_{2|1}(\cdot|s)$. The information matrix considered must be the joint distribution of both variables and it is the product of the known marginal and the aimed conditional $\xi_{12}(\cdot,\cdot) = \tilde{\xi}_1\xi_{2|1}(\cdot|s)$. Considering the typical optimization problem, now restricted to the knowledge of $\tilde{\xi}_1$, an optimal conditional design is obtained. For instance, if $s = 96.1$ the optimal conditional design for this type of units is

$$\xi^*(\cdot|s = 96.1) = \left\{ \begin{matrix} 0\% & 10\% & 20\% \\ 0.46 & 0.08 & 0.46 \end{matrix} \right\}.$$

Since they had used a specific design for this experiment, we were able to compute the efficiency of that design: 71.5%. This means the optimal design may save 28.5% of the experiments to obtain the same results. Table 6.3 shows some optimal percentages of additive given some initial densities. More details for this example can be found in López-Fidalgo et al. (2008a).

Table 6.3 A few values of the joint marginally restricted (MR) D-optimal design for uranium densification

Initial density	% additive	Initial density	% additive	Initial density	% additive
95.15	12.33	95.32	5.46	95.45	16.77
95.22	15.82	95.32	16.30	95.37	7.30
95.49	12.80	95.64	12.63	95.76	14.54
95.33	8.58	95.41	16.76	95.51	18.34
95.54	3.53	95.70	7.21	95.79	16.06
95.56	16.88	95.72	11.10	95.81	17.12
96.05	14.07	96.11	14.70	96.28	14.63
96.08	9.38	96.16	19.23	96.44	17.81
96.10	14.75	96.24	3.21	96.73	20.00
96.04	5.36	96.11	6.10	96.27	6.19
96.05	8.27	96.11	2.68	96.27	14.65

6.5 Marginally Restricted with Correlated Observations: Irish Wind Data

This case is related to a well-known dataset used by Gneiting (2002) to establish an appropriate correlation structure. Daily average wind speeds from 1961 to 1978, y, are measured in terms of elevations of $s = 11$ observation stations at different times, t. A simple linear model

$$E[y(s,t)] = 1 + \alpha s + \beta t$$

is considered. The marginal design of the different elevations is completely known, and the times for measuring have to be optimized. The marginal design of the 11 different elevations of these stations is known:

$$\tilde{\xi}_1 = \{10, 14, 20, 25, 41, 64, 69, 72, 85, 89, 104\}.$$

The objective is to obtain optimal times t for observations conditioned to particular elevations s. The design space is $\chi = \chi_1 \times \chi_2$, where $\chi_1 = \{10, 14, 20, 25, 41, 64, 69, 72, 85, 89, 104\}$, the actual possible elevations in meters, and $\chi_2 = [0, 30]$ measured in days. The covariance structure considered by Gneiting (2002) and Zhu and Stein (2005) is:

$$\operatorname{cov}(y, y') = \begin{cases} (0.901|t-t'|^{1.544}+1)^{-1} & \text{if } s = s', \\ 0.968(0.901|t-t'|^{1.544}+1)^{-1}\exp\left[-\frac{0.00134|s-s'|}{(0.901|t-t'|^{1.544}+1)^{\theta_2/2}}\right] & \text{if } s \neq s'. \end{cases}$$

They estimated the value of $\hat{\theta}_2 = 0.61$, which will be used here as known value of the parameter. Obtaining directly a MR D-optimal design for this case is computationally unavailable. Thus, an exchange algorithm (Brimkulov et al., 1986 and Ucinski & Atkinson, 2004 for an English version) will be adjusted to MR optimization.

Let $\tilde{\xi}_1 = \{s_1, \ldots, s_n\}$ be a marginal design. The objective is to find conditional designs $\xi_{2|1}(\cdot|s_i) = \{t_i\}, \quad i = 1, \ldots, n$ maximizing the determinant of the information matrix of the joint design. Let the covariance structure be $C(|s_i - s_j|, |t_i - t_j|, \theta_2)$. The parameter θ_2 will be assumed known, that is, there is no interest in estimating it. The information matrix whose determinant has to be maximized is then $M = X'\Sigma_Y^{-1}X$. The algorithm is described as follows:

1. Take an initial design, $\xi_{2|1}^{(0)}(\cdot|s_i) = \{t_i^0\}, \quad i = 1, \ldots, n$ with $|M| \neq 0$.
2. Let $\xi^{(l)}$ be the design obtained at stage l. For $I = \{1, \ldots, n\}$ compute $(i^*, t^*) = \arg\max_{(i,t)\in I\times\chi_2} \Delta(i,t)$, with

$$\Delta(i,t) = \frac{|M(\xi_{t_i \leftrightarrows t}^{(l)})| - |M(\xi^{(l)})|}{|M(\xi^{(l)})|}$$

where $t_i \leftrightarrows t$ means exchanging t_i with a general t.

Table 6.4 Joint optimal design for elevations and times

Elevations	10	14	20	25	41	64	69	72	85	89	104
Times	14.0	7.0	25.0	3.5	30.0	20.8	1.0	27.8	7.0	25.0	14.0

3. Let the new design $\xi^{(l+1)}$ be the same as $\xi^{(l)}$ except that $\xi^{(l)}_{2|1}(\cdot|s_{i^*}) = \{t^*\}$
4. Stop if $\Delta^* \le \delta$, where δ is some given positive tolerance.

The implementation details given by Ucinski and Atkinson, 2004 may be used here in a straightforward way. Here $n = 11$ and we have taken $\delta = 10^{-6}$ to stop the algorithm. Using as initial design the one given by the experimenters a determinant of 1.5471×10^8 was obtained. In eight iterations the following values of the determinant of the information matrix (divided by 10^8) were obtained sequentially: 2.1409, 2.5705, 2.8312, 3.0959, 3.1438, 3.1674, 3.1674, 3.1675. Table 6.4 shows the joint optimal design with an information of $|M| = 3.1675 \times 10^8$.

The optimal design is shown in Fig. 6.4. It can be seen that the uncorrelated case design is more extremal than the correlated one. This is a typical situation for correlated observations. An observation may have intrinsically more or less

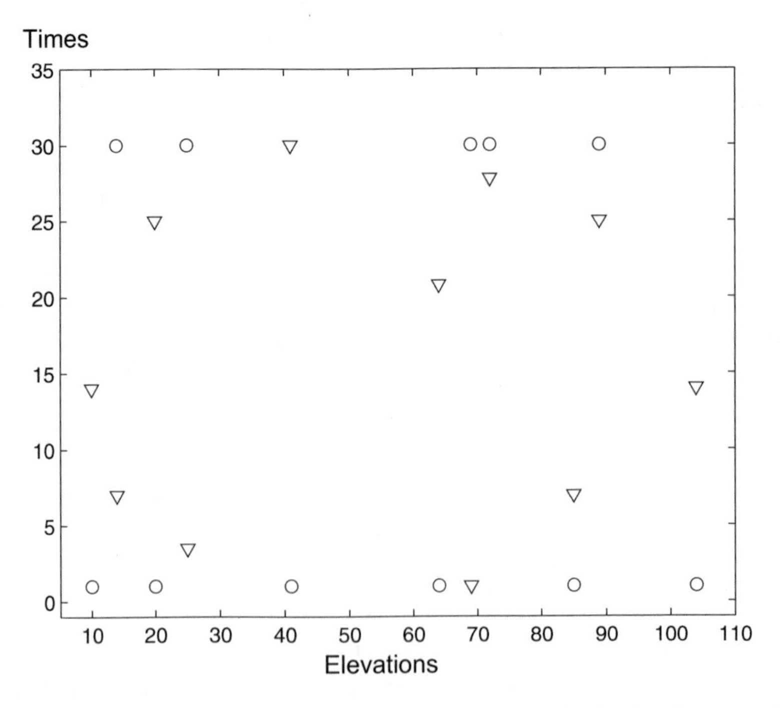

Fig. 6.4 Optimal points for correlated errors (O) compared to optimal points for uncorrelated errors (∇)

information about the observations around due to the correlation. Depending on the lower or higher correlation, this information influences the topology of the optimal design. More details for this example can be found in López-Fidalgo et al. (2008a).

6.6 Conditionally Restricted Designs: Prediction in Thoracic Surgery with Logistic Regression

In this section a more complex situation is considered where a conditional distribution could be assumed known as well in advance, apart from marginal distributions. Both types of variables may be present in a model (López-Fidalgo & Garcet-Rodríguez, 2004). They will be called marginally conditionally restricted (MCR) designs. This situation was motivated by a real case, which has been one of the most rewarding research experiences of the author of this book. This proves a real example is frequently so rich that very interesting new statistical methodology (including theoretical mathematics) has to be developed to tackle the problem. Varela et al. (2001) applied an exercise test to obtain more information to predict complications of surgery in the treatment of lung cancer. The authors considered the occurrence of any cardio-respiratory morbidity as a binary response variable, since its presence or absence is clinically associated to mortality, which is the most important outcome in major surgical procedures. The test consists in riding a static bicycle using a medical protocol. There are many independent variables but three are the most important. One is the "exercise time in minutes." The second one is the "expired volume of air in one second (Respiratory Function, RF)," measured as a percentage of the expected values for sex, age, and height. Values under the 25th percentile in the studied population have been considered pathological for the investigation purposes. The third variable is the "oxygen desaturation during the test." Here the first variable is completely under the control of the experimenter, the second variable is not subject to control, but its values are known before the exercise test is performed. As a part of routine medical evaluation before surgery, all the subjects have performed a test in which the expired lung volume is measured and recorded on patient's files. The last variable is not under control and the values are observed during the test. Oxygen amount (saturation) in blood depends on the physical condition of the subject. Absolute values are not relevant, for medical reasons; hence, the variable has been dichotomized according to whether desaturation (oxygen concentration under 90%) during exercise occurred. In this case the experiment has to be designed without knowing the values of this variable.

In what follows details of this problem are given. In particular, the exercise consists of riding a static bicycle using a medical protocol. The variables considered here are the "percentage of the normal value of volume of expired air for each subject" (x_1), "decrease of blood oxygen concentration during exercise under 90% during the exercise test" (x_2), and the "exercise time in minutes" (x_3). As was pointed out in the introduction, x_3 is completely under the control of the experimenter, x_1 is not subject to control, but its values are known before the exercise test is performed since it is recorded during routine preoperative tests. Variable x_2 is not under control and the occurrence of desaturation is observed during the exercise test. The objective was to predict the occurrence of any postoperative cardio-respiratory complication.

Let $\chi_1 \times \chi_2 \times \chi_3$ be the joint design space of $x^T = (x_1, x_2, x_3)$. The optimal design for a model of this kind yields a design on χ_2 to attain the best joint design on $\chi_1 \times \chi_2 \times \chi_3$, according to a particular criterion, subject to a specific marginal distribution on x_1 and a specific conditional distribution on x_2 given x_1 and x_3. These results would be useful when considering surgery. Since the response is binary in this case, a logistic model can be a good choice. Thus, the probability of $y = 1$ is

$$p(x, \theta) = \frac{1}{1 + e^{-\theta^T x}}.$$

The log-likelihood is then

$$\ell(\theta) = \log \frac{e^{-\theta^T x}}{1 + e^{-\theta^T x}} - y \log e^{-\theta^T x}.$$

Deriving the log-likelihood and computing the expectation, the Fisher Information Matrix for this model is obtained,

$$M(\xi, \theta) = E_{\xi,y} \left(\frac{\partial \ell(\theta)}{\partial \theta} \frac{\partial \ell(\theta)}{\partial \theta^T} \right)$$

$$= \int_\chi x^T x \frac{e^{\theta^T x}}{(1+e^{\theta^T x})^2} \xi(dx).$$

As mentioned in Chap. 3 for nonlinear models, the inverse of the Fisher Information Matrix is asymptotically proportional to the covariance of the MLE under regularity conditions (see Appendix B). This matrix depends on the parameters θ. If nominal values are available for the parameters, for example, from retrospective studies, then optimal design theory for linear models can be applied in this case. The design space, the nominal values of the parameters, and the restrictions are taken from Varela et al. (2001). In particular, $\chi_1 = \{0, 1\}$ with zero meaning a bad respiratory function ($RF \leq 52$, corresponding to the 25th percentile), $\chi_2 = \{0, 1\}$ where zero means that desaturation does not occur with a cut-off value of 90%, and $\chi_3 = \{12, 18\}$ being 12 and 18 minutes the standard times for the exercise. This categorization is the usual in the corresponding medical field.

The nominal values of the parameters and the initial joint design were obtained from Varela et al. (2001), $\theta^T = (1.7829, 0.2902, -0.3810)$ and

$$\xi^{(0)} = \left\{ \begin{array}{cccc} (0, 0, 12) & (0, 1, 12) & (1, 0, 12) & (1, 1, 12,) \\ 0.1522 & 0.0869 & 0.6957 & 0.0652 \end{array} \right\}.$$

From this design the following distributions are assumed to be known,

$$\tilde{\xi}_1 = \left\{ \begin{matrix} 0 & 1 \\ 0.2391 & 0.7609 \end{matrix} \right\},$$

that is, the sample is divided into two groups, one with about 24% of the patients with a low respiratory function ($RF \leq 52$) and the other group with about 76% of the patients with a high respiratory function. Also,

$$\tilde{\xi}_{2|13}(\cdot \mid 0, 12) = \left\{ \begin{matrix} 0 & 1 \\ 0.6366 & 0.3634 \end{matrix} \right\}, \quad \tilde{\xi}_{2|13}(\cdot \mid 1, 12) = \left\{ \begin{matrix} 0 & 1 \\ 0.9143 & 0.0857 \end{matrix} \right\}.$$

Since the 18-minute exercise was not considered in the experiment, the corresponding conditional designs were set up from the experience of the specialists,

$$\tilde{\xi}_{2|13}(\cdot \mid 0, 18) = \left\{ \begin{matrix} 0 & 1 \\ 0.4545 & 0.5455 \end{matrix} \right\}, \quad \tilde{\xi}_{2|13}(\cdot \mid 1, 18) = \left\{ \begin{matrix} 0 & 1 \\ 0.8714 & 0.1286 \end{matrix} \right\}.$$

It is usually feasible to find these numbers in practice from an experienced surgeon. The optimal design directly computed is

$$\left\{ \begin{matrix} (1,0,12) & (1,1,12) & (0,0,18) & (1,0,18) & (0,1,18) & (1,1,18) \\ 0.05357 & 0.005021 & 0.1087 & 0.61202 & 0.1304 & 0.09030 \end{matrix} \right\}.$$

The conditional designs to be performed in practice will be:

$$\xi_{3|1}(\cdot \mid 0) = \left\{ \begin{matrix} 18 \\ 1 \end{matrix} \right\}, \quad \xi_{3|1}(\cdot \mid 1) = \left\{ \begin{matrix} 12 & 18 \\ 0.07700 & 0.9230 \end{matrix} \right\}.$$

López-Fidalgo and Garcet-Rodríguez (2004) provided a rather general algorithm for computing these optimal designs. For D-optimality the algorithm has the following particular aspects:

- $x_3^{(n)}(x_1) = \arg\max_{x_3 \in \chi_3} \int_{\chi_2} x^T M^{-1}(\xi^{(n)}) x \, \tilde{\xi}_{2|13}(dx_2 \mid x_1, x_3)$.
- The procedure stops when

$$2 - \frac{1}{m} \int_{\chi_2 \times \chi_1} x^{(n)T} M^{-1}(\xi^{(n)}) x^{(n)} \, \tilde{\xi}_{2|13}(dx_2 \mid x_1, x_3^{(n)}(x_1)) \, \tilde{\xi}_1(dx_1) \geq \delta,$$

where $0 < \delta < 1$ is a lower bound for the efficiency and $x^{(n)}$ denotes here $(x_1, x_2, x_3^{(n)}(x_1))$.

After 11 iterations of the algorithm, an efficiency of more than 99% was reached for the design $\xi^{(11)}$:

$$\left\{\begin{array}{llllll} (0,0,12) & (1,0,12) & (0,1,12) & (1,1,12) & (0,0,18) & (1,0,18) \\ 0.006919 & 0.09487 & 0.003949 & 0.008892 & 0.1037 & 0.5727 \\ (0,1,18) & (1,1,18) & & & & \\ 0.1245 & 0.08449 & & & & \end{array}\right\}.$$

An efficiency of over 99.9% is obtained only after 100 iterations. Notice that the sum of the weights is not one because of the rounding-off during the computation process. It is preferable to round off the conditional design to the number of experiments to be performed in practice.

The optimal design dictates performing the exercise over 18 minutes with about 92.3% of the patients with $x_1 = 1$ and with all the patients with $x_1 = 0$. This means most of the patients are asked to do the hardest exercise for eighteen minutes, which is expected to be more informative than the 12-minute exercise. The design obtained with the algorithm is not optimal but has a high efficiency and allows the practitioner to choose about 4.55% of the patients with $RF \leq 52$ to perform the exercise over 12 minutes and the rest over 18 minutes.

The efficiency of the design used in Varela et al. (2001) is 65.9%, meaning that the D-optimal design saves about 34% of patients to achieve the same results. This efficiency can be lower if the design space considered is an interval of times $[0, A]$ with an appropriate A. There is not any medical experience at this point, but we have assumed the design space $[0, 20]$, which seems reasonable to the practitioners. The design $\tilde{\xi}_1$ will be the same and the conditional design $\tilde{\xi}_{2|13}$ is defined for general values $x_3 \in [0, 20]$ extrapolating the conditional designs the practitioners used for $x_3 = 12$ and 18,

$$\tilde{\xi}_{2|13}(\cdot \mid 0, x_3) = \left\{\begin{array}{cc} 0 & 1 \\ \frac{33-x_3}{33} & \frac{x_3}{33} \end{array}\right\}, \quad \tilde{\xi}_{2|13}(\cdot \mid 1, x_3) = \left\{\begin{array}{cc} 0 & 1 \\ \frac{140-x_3}{140} & \frac{x_3}{140} \end{array}\right\}.$$

Implementation of the algorithm becomes more complex. Starting with the same design as before and after eight iterations, an efficiency of over 96.8% was obtained adding two new points to the design, namely 11.16 and 11.90. Iteration 10 asks for the introduction of a new point, 12.75. Thus, it seems that forcing a two-point design at 12 and 20 could provide a highly efficient design. With this constraint after 27 iterations, an efficiency greater than 99.5% is obtained with the following design to be performed in practice,

$$\xi_{3|1}^{(27)}(\cdot \mid 0) = \left\{\begin{array}{cc} 12 & 20 \\ 0.01786 & 0.98214 \end{array}\right\}, \quad \xi_{3|1}^{(27)}(\cdot \mid 1) = \left\{\begin{array}{cc} 12 & 20 \\ 0.16071 & 0.83929 \end{array}\right\}.$$

This means choosing about 98.2% of the patients with $RF \leq 52$ and 83.9% of the patients with $RF > 52$ at random to perform the exercise over 20 minutes.

Table 6.5 Optimal design robustness against different true values of the parameters

$\theta_1 = 2,\ (\theta_2, \theta_3)$	$(0.1, -0.5)$	$(0.5, -0.5)$	$(0.5, -0.1)$	$(0.1, -0.1)$
Efficiency	0.9968	0.9972	0.9847	0.9835
$\theta_1 = 1,\ (\theta_2, \theta_3)$	$(0.1, -0.5)$	$(0.5, -0.5)$	$(0.5, -0.1)$	$(0.1, -0.1)$
Efficiency	0.9948	0.9951	0.9889	0.9885

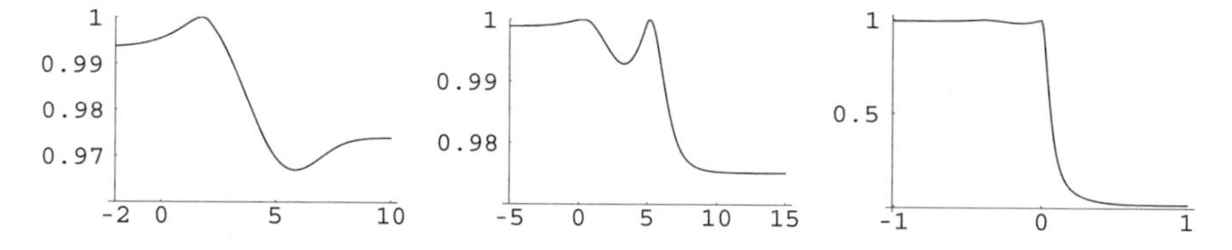

Fig. 6.5 Efficiencies of the optimal design for different true values of each of the three parameters (from left to right) fixing the other two at the nominal values

It is remarkable how augmenting the time to 20 minutes reduces the required experiments for the maximum time exercise. The efficiency of the Varela et al. (2001) design is now about 59.3%, indicating a considerable improvement.

Since nominal values of the parameters have been set up for the computation of the optimal design, a sensitivity analysis will help to measure the robustness of the optimal design with respect to possible true values of the parameters. Let $\xi^\star_{\theta_0}$ be the optimal design computed with the nominal values θ_0 and let $\xi^\star_\theta$ be the optimal design for the true values θ. The efficiency of $\xi^\star_{\theta_0}$ with respect to the true values is

$$\text{eff}_\theta(\xi^\star_{\theta_0}) = \left(\frac{|M_\theta(\xi^\star_{\theta_0})|}{|M_\theta(\xi^\star_\theta)|} \right)^{1/3}.$$

Table 6.5 shows high efficiencies for different possible true values near the nominal values of the parameters. Fixing true values of two parameters as the nominal values, a graphic of the efficiencies for different values of the third parameter provides a good picture of the sensitivity of the optimal design. Figure 6.5 shows high efficiencies, except for the case of positive true values of the third parameter.

6.7 Potential Censoring in the Design: The Complex Reality of Using an Optimal Design in Thoracic Surgery

In the previous section a good experimental design was found to predict cardiopulmonary morbidity after lung resection with standardized exercise oximetry. As mentioned above this could mean a significant save of experiments, that is, number of patients, for obtaining the same or better results. But realizing an optimal design in practice may involve new and complex situations. When the authors of this work approximated the physicians with the optimal design trying to convince then to use it new practical problems showed up. On the one hand, a 12-minute exercise is in the approved protocol for the trials. Asking patient to cycle more time is something new. We must take into account that some problem may show up during the exercise, and they actually happen from time to time, for example, a sudden stroke. Another degree of complexity, less traumatic, appears when a patient cannot complete the assigned experimental condition, for example, the prescribed exercise time. In the latter case the controlled variable has to be considered as potentially censored and thus the design can be censored (truncated). Then a known censoring probability distribution function has to be assumed for the controlled variable. Thus, when a particular design is tried, another different design is expected to happen according to this distribution. The information matrix of this expected design is the one to be used in the optimization problem.

Hackl (1995) provided a criterion based on D-optimality and obtained optimal exact uniform designs for possible missing observations in the quadratic model. Imhof et al. (2002, 2004) provided general procedures to compute approximate designs for this situation. The problem of potentially censored independent variables considered here is different. Garcet-Rodríguez et al. (2008) dealt with the problem of obtaining D-optimal approximate designs for a linear model when the values of some independent variables are potentially censored according to a known probability distribution function.

Here t is the time, that is going to be a variable potentially censored in a design space χ. The censoring distribution will be assumed known through a random variable T that measures the time a chosen experimental unit is going to stop given no prior limitation in time. In the real case mentioned above, T would be the time a generic patient stops if he starts to ride the bicycle without any time limit imposed in advance. Assume the censored time T has a probability distribution on a set, which includes the whole design space. Let $f(t)$ and $F(t)$ be the probability distribution function and the cumulative distribution function, respectively. A particular but typical case may be a distribution on $[0, \infty)$ with a design space contained in it.

Let $\hat{\xi}$ be the approximate design with finite support that is intended to be applied in practice. Then another design ξ is expected to result at the end of the experimentation. Therefore, a design $\hat{\xi}$ should be found such that the expected design ξ will be optimal. We will call an optimal design with this restriction censoring restricted (CER) optimal design. Sometimes it is possible to find $\hat{\xi}$

such that the expected design ξ will be optimal according to the criterion without censoring. But frequently this is not the case and a restricted search has to be done. This happens mainly when there is an optimal time at the highest possible time value. As a matter of fact, if the censoring distribution is continuous this value will never be reached.

Let a discrete design space be $\chi = \{t_1, t_2, \ldots, t_n\}$, where $t_1 < \ldots < t_k < \ldots < t_n$. The censoring distribution will be considered as a discrete distribution on χ. The cumulative distribution function will be $F(t) = \sum_{i=1}^{k} f(t_i)$, $t_k \leq t < t_{k+1}$, $k = 1, \ldots, n$, where $f(t_i) = P(T = t_i)$, $i = 1, \ldots, n$. This case may correspond to an experiment where n stages have to be completed and an experimental unit may stop the experiment at any of these stages. Thus, $f(t_i)$ will be the probability to stop exactly at time t_i, that is, completing stage i. When a design $\hat{\xi}$ is tried in practice, an expected censored design ξ will be actually performed following the rule:

1. All the tries at t_1 will succeed; thus, all the weight given to t_1, $\hat{\xi}(t_1)$ will remain for ξ.
2. The number of the tries at time t_2, which will not succeed, that is, that will stop at time t_1, will be proportional to $f(t_1)$ and therefore the number of tries succeeding will be proportional to $1 - f(t_1)$. Thus, a proportion $f(t_1)\hat{\xi}(t_2)$ of the sample size will actually stop at t_1 and the rest $[1 - f(t_1)]\hat{\xi}(t_2)$ will reach the time challenge t_2.
3. Following the same reasoning there will be a proportion of tries at time t_3 that is expected to succeed, $[f(t_3) + \cdots + f(t_n)]\hat{\xi}(t_3)$; a proportion that will stop at time t_2, $f(t_2)\hat{\xi}(t_3)$; and a proportion that will stop at time t_1, $f(t_1)\hat{\xi}(t_3)$.

A similar argument is used for the rest of the times. Therefore,

$$\xi(t_k) = [1 - F(t_{k-1})]\hat{\xi}(t_k) + \sum_{i=k+1}^{n} \hat{\xi}(t_i)P(T = t_k) \tag{6.1}$$

$$= [1 - F_{k-1}]\hat{\xi}(t_k) + f(t_k)[1 - \hat{\Xi}_k], \; k = 1, \ldots, n-1, \tag{6.2}$$

and

$$\xi(t_n) = f(t_n)\hat{\xi}(t_n) = [1 - F_{n-1}]\hat{\xi}(t_n), \tag{6.3}$$

where $F_k \equiv F(t_k)$, $\hat{\Xi}_k \equiv \sum_{i=1}^{k} \hat{\xi}(t_i)$, $k = 1, \ldots, n-1$; $F_0 \equiv 0$ and $\hat{\Xi}_0 \equiv 0$.

By definition ξ is a probability measure and so it may be considered as a design. From the expressions above $\hat{\xi}$ may be worked out in function of ξ as described in what follows,

$$\begin{pmatrix} \hat{\xi}(t_1) \\ \hat{\xi}(t_2) \\ \cdots \\ \hat{\xi}(t_n) \end{pmatrix} = \begin{pmatrix} 1-F_0 & f(t_1) & f(t_1) & \cdots & f(t_1) \\ 0 & 1-F_1 & f(t_2) & \cdots & f(t_2) \\ \cdots & \cdots & \cdots & \cdots & \cdots \\ 0 & 0 & 0 & \cdots & f(t_n) \end{pmatrix}^{-1} \begin{pmatrix} \xi(t_1) \\ \xi(t_2) \\ \cdots \\ \xi(t_n) \end{pmatrix} \tag{6.4}$$

$$= \begin{pmatrix} \frac{1}{1-F_0} & \frac{1}{1-F_0} - \frac{1}{1-F_1} & \cdots & \frac{1}{1-F_0} - \frac{1}{1-F_1} & \frac{1}{1-F_0} - \frac{1}{1-F_1} \\ 0 & \frac{1}{1-F_1} & \cdots & \frac{1}{1-F_1} - \frac{1}{1-F_2} & \frac{1}{1-F_1} - \frac{1}{1-F_2} \\ \cdots & \cdots & \cdots & \cdots & \cdots \\ 0 & 0 & \cdots & \frac{1}{1-F_{n-2}} & \frac{1}{1-F_{n-2}} - \frac{1}{1-F_{n-1}} \\ 0 & 0 & \cdots & 0 & \frac{1}{1-F_{n-1}} \end{pmatrix} \begin{pmatrix} \xi(t_1) \\ \xi(t_2) \\ \cdots \\ \xi(t_{n-1}) \\ \xi(t_n) \end{pmatrix}$$

$$= \begin{pmatrix} \frac{1-\Xi_0}{1-F_0} - \frac{1-\Xi_1}{1-F_1} \\ \frac{1-\Xi_1}{1-F_1} - \frac{1-\Xi_2}{1-F_2} \\ \cdots \\ \frac{1-\Xi_{n-2}}{1-F_{n-2}} - \frac{1-\Xi_{n-1}}{1-F_{n-1}} \\ \frac{\xi(t_n)}{f(t_n)} \end{pmatrix},$$

where $\Xi_k \equiv \sum_{i=1}^{k} \xi(t_i)$, $k = 1, \ldots, n-1$ and $\Xi_0 \equiv 0$.

The measure constructed in this way may not be a probability measure, and therefore, it cannot always be considered as an experimental design. It sums up to one, but the values are nonnegative if and only if,

$$\frac{1-\Xi_{i-1}}{1-F_{i-1}} \geq \frac{1-\Xi_i}{1-F_i}, \quad i = 1, \ldots, n-1. \tag{6.5}$$

that is, the ratio $r_i = (1-\Xi_i)/(1-F_i)$ is nonincreasing for $i = 1, \ldots, n-1$. Taking into account that the weights obtained sum up to 1, if this is satisfied the values have to be no greater than 1. Therefore, this is the condition for $\hat{\xi}$ to be an experimental design. Let $\Im_F$ be the set of these designs,

$$\Im_F = \{\xi \mid \xi \text{ satisfies (6.5)}\}.$$

Theorem 6.1 *The set $\Im_F$ is convex.*

Proof Let $\xi^{(1)}, \xi^{(2)} \in \Im_F, \alpha \in (0, 1)$ and $\xi = (1-\alpha)\xi^{(1)} + \alpha\xi^{(2)}$. With the notation used above,

$$1 - \Xi_i = \xi_{i+1} + \cdots + \xi_n = (1-\alpha)(\xi_{i+1}^{(1)} + \cdots + \xi_n^{(1)}) + \alpha(\xi_{i+1}^{(2)} + \cdots + \xi_n^{(2)})$$
$$= (1-\alpha)(1 - \Xi_i^{(1)}) + \alpha(1 - \Xi_i^{(2)}).$$

Therefore,

$$(1 - \Xi_i)(1 - F_{i-1}) = [(1-\alpha)(1 - \Xi_i^{(1)}) + \alpha(1 - \Xi_i^{(2)}](1 - F_{i-1})$$
$$\geq [(1-\alpha)(1 - \Xi_{i-1}^{(1)}) + \alpha(1 - \Xi_{i-1}^{(2)})](1 - F_i) = (1 - \Xi_{i-1})(1 - F_i).$$

□

From Theorem 1 of López–Fidalgo and Garcet–Rodríguez (2004), an equivalence theorem may be stated.

Theorem 6.2 *If Φ is a convex criterion function, then the following statements are equivalent:*

1. $\Phi[M(\xi^\star)] = \inf_{\xi \in \Im_F} \Phi[M(\xi)]$, *where $\xi^\star$ is the CER Φ-optimal design.*
2. $\inf_{N \in \mathbf{M}_F} \partial\Phi[M(\xi^\star), N] = \sup_{\xi \in \Im_F^+} \inf_{N \in \mathbf{M}_F} \partial\Phi[M(\xi), N]$, *where* $\mathbf{M}_F = \{M(\xi) \mid \xi \in \Im_F\}$ *and $\Im_F^+$ is the set of the designs with nonsingular information matrix.*
3. $\inf_{N \in \mathbf{M}_F} \partial\Phi[M(\xi^\star), N] = 0.$

The procedure to compute Φ-optimal designs under this restriction is as follows:

1. Compute the Φ-optimal design without any restriction, say ξ^*. If r_i^* is increasing for $i = 1, \ldots, n-1$, then compute $\hat{\xi}$ using Eq. (6.4) and the problem is solved. Otherwise go to step 2.
2. An optimal expected design subject to the restriction (6.5) must be found. The information matrix associated to a generic expected design ξ, obtained with Eqs. (6.2) and (6.3), is

$$M(\xi) = \sum_{k=1}^{n} \hat{\xi}(t_k) \left[\sum_{i=1}^{k-1} f(t_i)\eta(t_i)\eta^T(t_i) + (1 - F_{k-1})\eta(t_k)\eta^T(t_k) \right].$$

   The objective is then,

$$\xi_F^* = \arg\min\{\Phi[M(\xi)] \mid \xi \in \Im_F\}.$$

3. In any of the two cases the design to be used in practice has to be computed from the optimal expected design using formula (6.4).

Remark 6.1 A one-point design, say ξ_{t_k}, is in $\Im_F$ if and only if $F_{k-1} = 0$. A two-point design, say ξ_{t_k,t_j}, $k < j$, is in $\Im_F$ if and only if $F_{k-1} = 0$, $F_{j-1} = f_k\, \xi(t_k) \leq \frac{1-F_k}{1-F_{k-1}}$. There is not a way to find a simple rule for the rest of the cases. Thus, it is not possible to find simple generators of the set of CER designs.

Example 6.1 Let a model be,

$$\mathrm{E}(y) = \alpha_1 + \alpha_2 t,\ \mathrm{Var}(y) = \sigma^2,\ t \in \chi = \{0, 1, 2, 3\}.$$

Assume there is a binomial censoring distribution on χ, Bi(3, 1/3),

$$f \equiv \left\{ \begin{matrix} 0 & 1 & 2 & 3 \\ 1/27 & 2/9 & 4/9 & 8/27 \end{matrix} \right\}.$$

A general design

$$\xi \equiv \left\{ \begin{matrix} 0 & 1 & 2 & 3 \\ 1-p-q-r & p & q & r \end{matrix} \right\}$$

satisfies (6.5) if the sequence

$$\frac{1-\Xi}{1-F} \equiv \left\{ \frac{27(p+q+r)}{26}, \frac{27(q+r)}{20}, \frac{27r}{8} \right\},$$

is non increasing, that is, $10p - 3q - 3r \geq 0$ and $2q - 3r \geq 0$. The information matrix for this design is

$$M(\xi) = \begin{pmatrix} 1 & p+2q+3r \\ p+2q+3r & p+4q+9r \end{pmatrix}.$$

Maximizing the determinant subject to those restrictions, the CER D-optimal design will be,

$$\xi = \left\{ \begin{matrix} 0 & 1 & 2 & 3 \\ 71/162 & 7/54 & 7/27 & 14/81 \end{matrix} \right\}$$

with determinant $49/36$. It is well-known that the unrestricted D-optimal design for this model gives half of the weight to each extreme point 0 and 3. Its determinant is $9/4$ and the efficiency of the restricted optimal with respect to the unrestricted optimal is then $\frac{49/36}{9/4} = 7/9$, that is, 77.8%.

Once the optimal expected design ξ is computed, there is the way back to compute the design to be tried in practice $\hat{\xi}$,

$$\hat{\xi} = \left\{ \begin{array}{cccc} 0 & 1 & 2 & 3 \\ \frac{1-\Xi_0}{1-F_0} - \frac{1-\Xi_1}{1-F_1} & \frac{1-\Xi_1}{1-F_1} - \frac{1-\Xi_2}{1-F_2} & \frac{1-\Xi_2}{1-F_2} - \frac{1-\Xi_3}{1-F_3} & \frac{\xi(t_4)}{f(t_4)} \end{array} \right\}$$

$$= \left\{ \begin{array}{cccc} 0 & 1 & 2 & 3 \\ 1 - \frac{p+q+r}{26/27} & \frac{p+q+r}{26/27} - \frac{q+r}{20/27} & \frac{q+r}{20/27} - \frac{r}{8/27} & \frac{r}{8/27} \end{array} \right\} = \left\{ \begin{array}{cc} 0 & 3 \\ 5/12 & 7/12 \end{array} \right\}.$$

This result is quite meaningful since this is the safest way to get something as similar as possible to the unrestricted optimal design.

Example 6.2 Let another model be

$$E(y) = \alpha_1 + \alpha_2 t + \alpha_3 t^2, \ \mathrm{Var}(y) = \sigma^2, \ t \in \chi = [0, 1].$$

In this case exponential censoring is assumed,

$$G(t) = -e^{-t} \begin{pmatrix} 1 & 1+t & 2+2t+t^2 \\ 1+t & 2+2t+t^2 & 6+6t+3t^2+t^3 \\ 2+2t+t^2 & 6+6t+3t^2+t^3 & 24+24t+12t^2+4t^3+t^4 \end{pmatrix}.$$

Let an arbitrary design be

$$\hat{\xi} = \left\{ \begin{array}{ccc} 0 & 0.513 & 1 \\ 0.254 & 0.120 & 0.626 \end{array} \right\}.$$

Then, the design expected to happen is

$$\xi(t) = \begin{cases} 0.254 & \text{if } t = 0, \\ 0.120e^{-t} & \text{if } 0 < t < 0.513, \\ 0.120e^{-0.254} & \text{if } t = 0.513, \\ 0.746e^{-t} & \text{if } 0.513 < t < 1, \\ 0.626e^{-1} & \text{if } t = 1. \end{cases}$$

The efficiencies of $\hat{\xi}$ and ξ with respect to the D-optimal unrestricted design are 80.1% and 89.7%, respectively.

6.8 Censoring in the Response

Let $h(t|\theta, z)$ be the pdf of failure time (time to event) t and $z \in \chi$ be the design variable. Let $\theta = (\theta_1, \ldots, \theta_k)$ be unknown parameters to be estimated. Let $[0, b]$ be the period of the study and assume there is a random arrival of unit i at time I_i. The maximum possible time in the study is $c_i = b - I_i$, assuming there is right censoring.

Example 6.3 Let us assume the most simple case of designing two treatments, that is, $\chi = \{0, 1\}$, and let consider the model $t \equiv \mathcal{E}(\alpha + \beta z)$. Let $h(t) = (\alpha + \beta z)e^{-(\alpha+\beta z)t}$ be the pdf. Then the survival function is $S(t) = e^{-(\alpha+\beta z)t}$.

The conditional probability density function of the times observed x_i given c_i is

$$g_{x|c}(x_i|c_i; z_i, \alpha, \beta) =$$

$$= \begin{cases} f(x_i) = (\alpha + \beta z_i)e^{-(\alpha+\beta z_i)x_i} & \text{if } x_i < c_i, \\ S(x_i) = e^{-(\alpha+\beta z_i)c_i} & \text{if } x_i = c_i. \end{cases}$$

If $\tilde{\xi}_1(c)$ is the marginal pdf of the maximum possible time c then the joint pdf of (x_i, c_i) is

$$g(x_i, c_i; z_i, \alpha, \beta) = g_{x|c}(x_i|c_i; z_i, \alpha, \beta) \cdot \tilde{\xi}_1(c),$$

whose logarithm is

$$\ell(\alpha, \beta) = \log \tilde{\xi}_1(c) + \begin{cases} \log(\alpha + \beta z_i) - (\alpha + \beta z_i)x_i & \text{if } x_i < c_i, \\ -(\alpha + \beta z_i)c_i & \text{if } x_i = c_i. \end{cases}$$

Thus, the FIM at (c, z) is

$$I(c, z) = \mathrm{E}\left(-\frac{\partial^2 L(\alpha, \beta)}{\partial(\alpha, \beta)^2}\right) = \frac{1 - e^{-(\alpha+\beta z)c}}{(\alpha + \beta z)^2}\begin{pmatrix} 1 & z \\ z & z^2 \end{pmatrix}.$$

The aim is a conditional design

$$\xi_{2|1}(z|c) = \begin{Bmatrix} 0 & 1 \\ 1 - p(c) & p(c) \end{Bmatrix}$$

such that $\xi(c, z) = \xi_{2|1}(z|c) \cdot \tilde{\xi}_1(c)$ is optimal.

Table 6.6 Optimal design for different nominal values of the parameters

α	0.1	0.1	0.1	10	10	10	100	100	100
β	0.1	10	100	0.1	10	100	0.1	10	100
c^*	0.70	0.61	0.58	0.55	0.53	0.51	0.51	0.51	0.50

If a linear model with regressors $(w(c, z),\ w(c, z)\, z)$, $w(c, z) = \sqrt{\frac{1-e^{-(\alpha+\beta z)c}}{(\alpha+\beta z)^2}}$ is considered with a uniform marginal distribution $\tilde{\xi}_1(c) = \mathcal{U}[0, 1]$, then the optimal conditional design (on c) is $z^* = 1$ for $c < c^*$ and $z^* = 0$ for $c > c^*$, where $c^\star$ is given in Table 6.6.

López-Fidalgo et al. (2009), López-Fidalgo and Rivas-López (2014), Konstantinou et al. (2013a), Konstantinou et al. (2013b), Rivas-López et al. (2014) considered this and more complex cases of censoring in the response variable.

Appendix A
Some Mathematical Concepts and Properties

1. **Convexity of the logarithm of the inverse of the determinant:**
   Let $M = (1-\alpha)M_1 + \alpha M_2$ with M_1 and M_2 positive definite matrices, then $|M| \geq |M_1|^{1-\alpha}|M_2|^{\alpha}$ (see, e.g., Beckenbach & Bellman, 1965). Therefore, $\log|M| \geq (1-\alpha)\log|M_1| + \alpha\log|M_2|$ and then $-\log|M|$ is a convex function.
2. Let A and B be two nonsingular squared matrices such that $A+B$ is nonsingular, then

$$(A+B)^{-1} = A^{-1} - A^{-1}B\left(I + A^{-1}B\right)^{-1}A^{-1}.$$

3. Let a symmetrical matrix be defined by blocks,

$$M = \begin{pmatrix} A & B \\ B^T & C \end{pmatrix},$$

   then, assuming all are invertible,

$$M^{-1} = \begin{pmatrix} (A - BC^{-1}B^T)^{-1} & -AB(C - B^TA^{-1}B)^{-1} \\ -(C - B^TA^{-1}B)^{-1}B^TA & (C - B^TA^{-1}B)^{-1} \end{pmatrix},$$

$$\det M = \det A \det(C - B^TA^{-1}B) = \det C \det(A - BC^{-1}B^T).$$

4. Let A and B be positive definite matrices and $\alpha \in [0, 1]$, then

$$[\alpha A + (1-\alpha)B]^{-1} \leq \alpha A^{-1} + (1-\alpha)B^{-1}.$$

5. The *generalized inverse (g-inverse)* or *pseudo-inverse* of any matrix A of dimension $\nu_1 \times \nu_2$, square or not, singular or not, is a class of matrices A^- such that $AA^-A = A$. In this book just symmetric matrices are of interest. Let A be a symmetric matrix, then it has always a generalized inverse and

J. López-Fidalgo, *Optimal Experimental Design*, Lecture Notes in Statistics 226,
https://doi.org/10.1007/978-3-031-35918-7

it is unique just in the case of a nonsingular matrix, which is the inverse. The matrix A defines a linear function assigning vector u to vector Au. Let $\mathrm{Img}(A) = \{Au \mid u \in \mathbb{R}^{\nu_2}\}$ and $\mathrm{Ker}(A) = \{u \in \mathbb{R}^{\nu_2} \mid Au = 0\}$ the image and kernel of the linear function generated by A. It is well-known that $\mathrm{Img}(A)$ and $\mathrm{Ker}(A)$ are orthogonal subspaces and the union generates $\mathbb{R}^m$. These are some other properties:

(a) A^- is a g-inverse if and only if $AA^-u = u$ for every $u \in \mathbb{R}$.
(b) If $\mathrm{Img}(H) \subset \mathrm{Img}(A)$, then $H^T A^- H$ is unique.

Proof For every $u \in \mathbb{R}$ there exists $w \in \mathbb{R}$ such that $H^T u = Aw$. Therefore,

$$u^T H A^- H^T u = w^T A A^- A w = w^T A w.$$

This happens for any vector u and any g-inverse A^-; thus, HA^-H^T does not depend on the choice of A^-. □

Appendix B
Linear Models

Let y be a univariate response and assume x is a vector of explanatory variables (predictors), which can be controlled by the experimenter. A *linear model* trying to describe the relationship between y and the values of x, or better the influence of x on y, can be described as

$$y = \theta^T f(x) + \varepsilon, \tag{B.1}$$

where $\theta^T = (\theta_1, \ldots, \theta_m)$ is the vector of unknown parameters to be estimated, $f^T(x) = (f_1(x), \ldots, f_m(x))$ is a vector of known linearly independent continuous functions, usually called *regressors*, and x is a nonrandom experimental condition. The response y is assumed *normal* with mean $\mathrm{E}(y) = \theta^T f(x)$, that is, $\mathrm{E}(\varepsilon) = 0$ and constant unknown variance $\mathrm{var}(y) = \mathrm{var}(\varepsilon) = \sigma^2$. The latter property is called *homoscedasticity*. Moreover, all the observations (experiments) are assumed *independent*. Some examples with this notation are given in 2.1.

Thus, a linear model assumes independence, normality, homoscedasticity, as well as linearity of the mean with respect to the parameters.

Assume the experiments are realized n times at n *experimental conditions* $x_1, x_2, \ldots, x_n$. Let $y_1, y_2, \ldots, y_n$ be the corresponding independent outcomes (responses) and $\varepsilon_1, \varepsilon_2, \ldots, \varepsilon_n$ the random errors, then

$$X = \begin{pmatrix} f_1(x_1) & \cdots & f_m(x_1) \\ \cdots & \cdots & \cdots \\ \cdots & f_i(x_j) & \cdots \\ \cdots & \cdots & \cdots \\ f_1(x_n) & \cdots & f_m(x_n) \end{pmatrix}, \; Y = \begin{pmatrix} y_1 \\ \vdots \\ y_i \\ \vdots \\ y_n \end{pmatrix}, \; \mathcal{E} = \begin{pmatrix} \varepsilon_1 \\ \vdots \\ \varepsilon_i \\ \vdots \\ \varepsilon_n \end{pmatrix},$$

J. López-Fidalgo, *Optimal Experimental Design*, Lecture Notes in Statistics 226,
https://doi.org/10.1007/978-3-031-35918-7

and (B.1) can be expressed in matrix form as

$$Y = X\theta + \mathcal{E}.$$

Remark B.1 In the literature of linear models $f_j(x_i)$ is frequently denoted as x_{ij}. Notation $f_j(x_i)$ refers directly to the design space where the x_i are selected, what is more convenient for experimental design purposes.

Theorem B.1 *For linear models the Least Squares Estimators (LSEs) coincide with the Maximum Likelihood Estimators.*

Proof Let X_j be the j-th column of X, corresponding to regressor j ($j = 1, \ldots, m$). Denote the mean of the components of X_j by $\bar{x}_j$ and $\bar{X}_j^T = (\bar{x}_j, \ldots, \bar{x}_j)$. Then $X_j - \bar{X}_j$. $j = 1, \ldots, m$ are vectors with zero mean. If the components of these vectors are small in absolute value, then the dispersion is small. The ordinary norm in $\mathbb{R}^n$ is defined as

$$||X_j - \bar{X}_j||^2 = \sum_{i=1}^{n} (x_{ij} - \bar{x}_j)^2.$$

The angle, α, between two vectors gives an idea of its relationship through the scalar product,

$$(X_j - \bar{X}_j)^T (X_{j'} - \bar{X}_{j'}) = \sum_i (x_{ij} - \bar{x}_j)(x_{ij'} - \bar{x}_{j'})$$
$$= ||X_j - \bar{X}_j|| \cdot ||X_{j'} - \bar{X}_{j'}|| \cos\alpha_{jj'}.$$

As a matter of fact,

$$\cos\alpha_{jj'} = \frac{(X_j - \bar{X}_j)^T (X_{j'} - \bar{X}_{j'})}{||X_j - \bar{X}_j|| \cdot ||X_{j'} - \bar{X}_{j'}||} = \frac{\text{cov}(X_j, X_{j'})}{\sqrt{\text{var}(X_j)\text{var}(X_{j'})}} = \text{corr}(X_j, X_{j'}),$$

where "cov," "var," and "corr" stand here for sample covariance, variance, and correlation between two variables, respectively. Thus, geometrical orthogonality means uncorrelation. We look for an estimator $\hat{\theta}$ such that the distance between the vectors of the responses and the predictions made with $\hat{\theta}$, say $\hat{Y} = X\hat{\theta}$, is minimum,

$$||\mathcal{E}||^2 = ||Y - \hat{Y}||^2 = ||Y - X\hat{\theta}||^2.$$

This is by definition the least squares method. Let E_X be the linear subspace of $\mathbb{R}^n$ generated by the vectors X_j, $j = 1, \ldots, m$. Since $\mathcal{E} = Y - \hat{Y}$ and $\hat{Y} = X\hat{\theta} \in E$ then the norm of $\mathcal{E}$ is minimized when E and $\mathcal{E}$ are orthogonal, that is, when the generators of E and $\mathcal{E}$ are orthogonal (null scalar product),

$$X_j^T \mathcal{E} = 0, \; j = 1, \ldots, m.$$

That is,

$$0 = X^T \mathcal{E} = X^T (Y - X\hat{\theta}),$$

and then

$$\hat{\theta} = (X^T X)^{-1} X^T Y.$$

Using the properties of the covariance matrix of a linear transformation, the covariance matrix of the estimators is then

$$\Sigma_{\hat{\theta}} = (X^T X)^{-1}.$$

Let us compute now the MLE assuming normality. The log-likelihood function is then

$$\ell(\theta) = -\frac{n}{2} \log(2\pi\sigma^2) - \frac{1}{2\sigma^2}(Y - X\theta)^T (Y - X\theta).$$

Optimizing the second term gives the LSE. They will be computed here differentiating with respect to θ and finding the roots of the so-called likelihood equation,

$$\frac{\partial \ell(\theta)}{\partial \theta} = -\frac{1}{2\sigma^2} X^T (Y - X\theta) = 0,$$

then

$$\hat{\theta} = (X^T X)^{-1} X^T Y,$$

that are the LSE previously computed. □

Remark B.2

1. Additionally, the MLE of σ can also be computed, while there is not LSE for it,

$$\frac{\partial \ell(X, \theta)}{\partial (\sigma^2)} = -\frac{n}{2\sigma^2} + \frac{1}{2\sigma^4}(Y - X\theta)^T (Y - X\theta) = 0,$$

   then

$$\hat{\sigma^2} = \frac{1}{n}(Y - X\hat{\theta})^T (Y - X\hat{\theta}).$$

2. This procedure is actually the projection of vector Y on the subspace E_X, giving $\hat{Y} = X\hat{\theta} = X(X^T X)^{-1} X^T Y$. The *projector matrix* is therefore $P = X(X^T X)^{-1} X^T$.

3. If the observations are correlated with covariance matrix Σ_Y known, all the results of the theorem are valid if the distance is transformed by this matrix,

$$||Y - \hat{Y}||_{\Sigma_Y^{-1}} = X^T \Sigma_Y^{-1} \mathcal{E},$$

and therefore

$$\hat{\theta} = (X^T \Sigma_Y^{-1} X)^{-1} X^T \Sigma_Y^{-1} Y,$$
$$\Sigma_{\hat{\theta}} = (X^T \Sigma_Y^{-1} X)^{-1}.$$

The LSEs have an important property even without the normality assumption. This is given by the celebrated Gauss–Markov theorem. Under some mild conditions the LSEs are the *Best Linear Unbiased Estimators* (BLUEs), where the meaning of these words is

Linear estimator: $\tilde{\theta} = CY$, for a matrix C independent of θ, but dependent on X.
Unbiased estimator: $\mathrm{E}(\tilde{\theta}) = \theta$.
Best: "Minimizing" the Mean Squared Error (MSE), $\mathrm{E}[(\tilde{\theta} - \theta)(\tilde{\theta} - \theta)^T]$. If the estimator is unbiased, then $\mathrm{E}[(\tilde{\theta} - \theta)(\tilde{\theta} - \theta)^T] = \Sigma_{\tilde{\theta}}$. Since they are matrices, "minimizing" means that $\Sigma_{\hat{\theta}} \leq \Sigma_{\tilde{\theta}}$ for any linear unbiased estimator $\tilde{\theta}$. The inequality is in the Loewner sense, that is, $\Sigma_{\hat{\theta}} - \Sigma_{\tilde{\theta}}$ is nonnegative definite.

Theorem B.2 (Gauss–Markov) *The LSEs are the BLUEs if the following conditions are satisfied:*

(i) The explanatory variables are nonrandom.
(ii) $E(\varepsilon_i) = 0,\ i = 1, \ldots, n.$
(iii) $var(\varepsilon_i) = \sigma^2,\ i = 1, \ldots, n$ *(heteroscedasticity).*
(iv) $corr(\varepsilon_i, \varepsilon_i') = 0,\ i \neq i'$ *(uncorrelated observations).*

Proof Let $\tilde{\theta} = WY$ be a linear estimator and define $D = W - (X^T X)^{-1} X^T$. The estimator $\tilde{\theta}$ is unbiased if

$$\begin{aligned}\theta = \mathrm{E}(\tilde{\theta}) &= \mathrm{E}\{[(X^T X)^{-1} X^T + D](X\theta + \varepsilon)\} = [(X^T X)^{-1} X^T + D] X\theta \\ &= (I + D)X\theta.\end{aligned}$$

Then $DX = 0$ and the covariance matrix of the estimators is

$$\begin{aligned}\Sigma_{\hat{\theta}} &= W \Sigma_Y W^T \\ &= \sigma^2 W W^T \\ &= \sigma^2 [(X^T X)^{-1} X^T + D][(X^T X)^{-1} X^T + D]^T\end{aligned}$$

$$= \sigma^2[(X^TX)^{-1} + (X^TX)^{-1}X^TD^T + DX(X^TX)^{-1} + DD^T]$$
$$= \sigma^2(X^TX)^{-1} + \sigma^2DD^T.$$

and therefore $\Sigma_{\hat{\theta}} - \sigma^2(X^TX)^{-1} = DD^T \geq 0.$ □

Remark B.3 Gauss–Markov theorem is still valid if the observations are correlated with potential different variances. The proof is similar including the covariance matrix Σ_Y appropriately.

Corollary B.1 *If $c \in E_X$, where E_X is the linear subspace of $\mathbb{R}^m$ generated by the columns of X, then $c^T\theta$ is estimable, $c^T\hat{\theta}$ is BLUE, and the variance is $\sigma^2c^T(X^TX)^{-1}c$. In particular, if $c^T = (0\ldots0, 1, 0\ldots0)$ we have the estimator of a particular parameter.*

B.1 Useful Results for Nonlinear Models

The convergence of the MLEs to the normal distribution and to the bound of the celebrated *Cramér-Rao theorem* gives an important result which makes the optimal design theory for linear models applicable to general statistical models.

Theorem B.3 (Cramér-Rao) *Let $h(y, x; \theta)$ be a parametric family of pdfs, from absolute continuous or discrete distributions, defining a statistical model. Let $T(X)$ be an estimator of θ and assume the following regularity conditions are satisfied:*

(i) For every possible (y, x) such that $h(y, x; \theta) > 0$, the score

$$\frac{\partial \log h(y, x; \theta)}{\partial \theta}$$

exists and all the components are finite.

(ii) The operations of integration with respect to x and differentiation with respect to θ can be interchanged in the expectation of T,

$$\frac{\partial}{\partial \theta}\int T(x)\,h(y, x; \theta)dy = \int T(x)\,\frac{\partial}{\partial \theta}h(y, x; \theta)dy.$$

whenever the second term is finite.

Let

$$M_\theta = E_h\left[\frac{\partial \log h(y, x; \theta)}{\partial \theta^T}\,\frac{\partial \log h(y, x; \theta)}{\partial \theta^T}\right] = -E_h\left[\frac{\partial^2 \log h(y, x; \theta)}{\partial \theta^2}\right]$$

be the Fisher Information Matrix. Let T be an estimator of θ with expected value $\omega(\theta) = E_h(T)$. Then

$$\Sigma_T \geq \frac{\partial \omega(\theta)}{\partial \theta} M_\theta^{-1} \frac{\partial \omega(\theta)}{\partial \theta^T},$$

with the Loewner ordering.

Remark B.4

1. If the estimate is unbiased, $\omega(\theta) = \theta$, then $\Sigma_T \geq M_\theta^{-1}$ with the Loewner ordering.
2. Condition (ii) of the theorem is satisfied if one of the following conditions holds,
   - Function h is bounded for y and the support of y does not depend on θ.
   - Function h is continuously differentiable on θ and its integral converges for every θ.
3. The bound is reached asymptotically for the MLEs. In particular, under regularity conditions,

$$\sqrt{n}(\hat{\theta} - \theta) \xrightarrow{L} \mathcal{N}\left(0, M_\theta^{-1}\right).$$

   This is just valid for uncorrelated observations since the proof is based on the Central Limit Theorem. Some authors study conditions where the inverse of the FIM can be used to approximate the covariance matrix for correlated observations, such as Pázman (2004, 2007). There is a kind of Central Limit Theorem for weak correlation that can also be considered here. In any case what is needed for using the optimal design theory for correlated observations is that the criterion is monotonic for actual covariance matrices with respect to the corresponding FIMs. That is, if there is an improvement of the FIM from a step to the next in the algorithm, then there is also an improvement in the covariance matrix, according to the criterion. This should happen monotonically, at least in trend.

B.2 Confidence Regions

The confidence ellipsoid of the parameters comes from this matrix,

$$(\hat{\theta} - \theta)^T (X^T X)^{-1} (\hat{\theta} - \theta) \leq m F_{m,n-m,\gamma} S_R^2,$$

where $F_{m,n-m,\gamma}$ stands for the quantile γ (confidence level) of the F-distribution; $S_R^2 = \frac{1}{n-m} \sum_{i=0}^{n} e_i^2$ is the residual variance; and $\mathcal{E} = Y - X\hat{\theta} = (e_1, \ldots, e_n)^T$ are the residuals.

The confidence band for the mean at a particular value is

$$y_{m,i} = \hat{y}_{m,i} \pm t_{n-m,\frac{\gamma+1}{2}} S_R \sqrt{X_i^T (X^T X)^{-1} X_i},$$

where X_i^T is the i-th row of X.

The individual prediction band for a particular response at specific conditions is

$$y_i = \hat{y}_i \pm t_{n-m,\frac{\gamma+1}{2}} S_R \sqrt{1 + X_i^T (X^T X)^{-1} X_i}.$$

Appendix C
Analysis of the Variance and Classical Experimental Design

In this introduction to linear models the case of categorical explanatory variables is included, although the usual approach is slightly different from that of regression. The aim is testing differences between the means of several groups. Thus, when the response variable is numerical and the explanatory variables are categorical, the linear models used receive the name of Analysis of the Variance (ANOVA). In Sect. 2.1 an example was shown to prove this is actually a linear model in the general sense introducing binary dummy variables. Most of the theory of design of experiments (DOE) has been formulated for this type of models looking for desirable properties of the experimental designs and providing particular designs, some of them with proper name, for different purposes or situations.

In this context the explanatory categorical variables are called *factors*. The possible values of a factor are called *levels* and they determine the different groups. Sometimes the levels are called *treatments* and the corresponding variable, *treatment factor*. Each factor provides a *way* of classification.

A general model can be defined as follows:

$$
\begin{aligned}
y_{ijk\ldots r} = \mu & \\
& +\alpha_i + \beta_j + \gamma_k + \ldots \text{(principal effects)} \\
& +(\alpha\beta)_{ij} + (\alpha\gamma)_{ik} + (\beta\gamma)_{jk} + \ldots \text{(order 2 interaction effects)} \\
& +(\alpha\beta\gamma)_{ijk} + \ldots \text{(order 3 interaction effects)} \\
& +\ldots \\
& +\varepsilon_{ijk\ldots r} \text{(random error + specification error)},
\end{aligned}
$$

where $\varepsilon_{ijk\ldots r} \sim \mathcal{N}(0, \sigma^2)$ are all independent. Subscript r stands for the replicates.

In this model α_i, $\beta_j \ldots$ are the *principal effects* of each level of each factor, while $(\alpha\beta)_{ij}$, $(\alpha\gamma)_{ik} \ldots$ are the *interaction effects* of order 2 and measure the effects in the response of the interaction of two factors. It is worth mentioning that

J. López-Fidalgo, *Optimal Experimental Design*, Lecture Notes in Statistics 226,
https://doi.org/10.1007/978-3-031-35918-7

$(\alpha\beta)_{ij} \neq \alpha_i \cdot \beta_j$, but a different parameter named with two letters between brackets. The concept of interaction does not mean a relationship between the two factors, but how their joint action affects the response. Interactions of any order can be considered in the same way, although the interpretation becomes harder and harder, and they are usually neglected in the model. In that case the effects discarded feed the error term.

The following constraints, or other of that kind, are needed, $\sum_i \alpha_i = 0$, $\sum_j \beta_j = 0$, $\sum_i (\alpha\beta)_{ij} = 0$, $\sum_j (\alpha\beta)_{ij} = 0, \ldots$ This means the effects are considered with respect to the global mean μ. Frequently, a basal level is considered as reference, for example, $\alpha_1 = 0$ or $(\alpha\beta)_{i1} = 0$ for all i. This is another alternative to the previous one.

The philosophy behind the analysis of these models is separating the *total variability* of the responses, no matter the group they come from, into the variability explained by the model, M, and the residual variability (Sum of the Square Errors) not explained by the model, E: $T = M + E$. The test for checking the model and so the hypothesis of the equality of the means of all the groups should be performed checking how large is M with respect to E by using the F probability distribution. The particular null hypotheses for principal and interaction effects would be

$$\begin{aligned} \mathrm{H}_0: \quad \alpha_i &= 0, \forall i, \\ \mathrm{H}_0: \quad \beta_j &= 0, \forall j, \\ \mathrm{H}_0: (\alpha\beta)_{ij} &= 0, \forall i, j, \\ \ldots \end{aligned}$$

All this procedure is summarized in the so-called ANOVA table. Table C.1 shows the case for a two-way model with interaction.

Once the ANOVA is performed the residuals should be used to check the basic assumptions of the model (*residual analysis*) of independence, normality and homoscedasticity. If the assumptions are satisfied and some tests are significant, then some post hoc analysis is usually needed to check the actual significant differences

Table C.1 ANOVA table for a two-way model with interaction

Source	SS	df	$MSS = \frac{SS}{df}$	$F = \frac{MSS}{S_R^2}$	p-value
Fact. A	A	$I-1$	S_A^2	F_A	$P(F_{I-1,g} > F_A)$
Fact. B	B	$J-1$	S_B^2	F_B	$P(F_{J-1,g} > F_B)$
Interact.	C	$(I-1)(J-1)$	S_C^2	F_C	$P(F_{(I-1)(J-1),g} > F_C)$
Model	$M = A + B + C$	$IJ-1$	S_M^2	F_M	$P(F_{IJ-1,g} > F_M)$
Resid.	E	$g = IJ(R-1)$	S_R^2		
Total	$T = M + E$	$IJR-1$			

that are of interest for the study. Deviations from the basic assumptions have more or less importance. In particular,

- Lack of normality is not an issue for large sample sizes.
- If the size of each group is about the same (largest size $\leq$ twice the smallest), heteroscedasticity does not affect much the test.
- Dependence of the observations has the worst consequences. This stresses the importance of randomizing and looking after a careful experimentation.

If the ANOVA cannot be performed in the present form, then some solutions are

- Transformations to reach normality and/or heteroscedasticity.
- Nonparametric tests instead of ANOVA. A typical one is the Kruskal–Wallis test.
- Model with a covariance structure to deal with correlated observations.

A *complete factorial design* is nothing else that all possible combinations of all the levels of all the factors in the model. The design can be completely or incompletely *replicated* a number of times. A *cell* is referred as the set of the observations of one of these combinations of levels. Having several observations in each cell allows for estimating the variance in each cell and then making inferences for all the parameters in the model, including *interactions* of two or more factors. Increasing the number of factors and levels, the number of combinations increases exponentially and sooner than later the number of experiments needed would be too large. Then *fractional factorial designs* are typically used in practice. An important part of the DOE theory is related to the appropriate choice of such a fraction of the complete design.

These are some types of designs:

- *Factorial and fractional designs*, which have already been mentioned.
- *Screening designs*: Select influential factors from a number of them, usually in an exploratory phase.
- *Nested or hierarchical designs*: The levels of the nested factor are different for each level of the parent factor (Fig. C.1). One example is the sector of the economy (primary, secondary, and tertiary) and then different areas of companies pending from each of these levels, such as fishing, farming, or mining for the primary sector or transport, entertainment, or consulting for the tertiary.
- *Split-plot designs* are used when the levels of some factors are difficult or more expensive to change and then each of them is fixed until all possible experiments for the possible levels of the easy-to-change factors are realized.

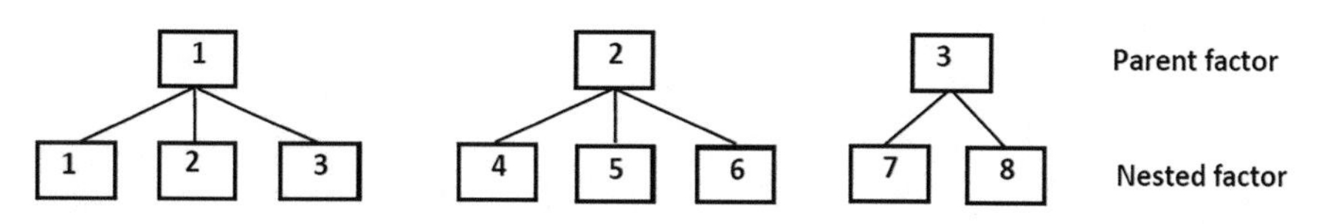

Fig. C.1 Nested design

Thus, the experiment is not randomized and the structure of it has to be taken into account in the analysis. The main treatments are called *Whole plot* while the remaining variables are the *Split-plot*. Random effects must be considered in this framework. A typical example is an oven that can heat several elements at the same time. For a strict randomization of the experiments, we should heat just one each time becoming more expensive and slow. Thus, using the corresponding correction and a random effects model, we can take advantage of heating several elements each time.

- *Sequential* and *adaptive* designs help to perform the right quantity of experiments, improving the design after having a new observation.
- *Response surface* designs are a particular case of sequential designs looking for the maximum or the minimum of some observable variable changing the values of the explanatory variables. In this case there is not a model and successive approximations by linear and quadratic models are made to check how far from the optimal we are and what the right direction to continue the search is.
- *Mixture experiments* are related to the optimal building of a new product composed by different possible proportions of elements. This is applied to the development of drugs, concrete, metals, fuel, perfumes ...

In the ANOVA framework the design is very much determined by the model and the design determines the model as well. A different approach, although complementary, is that of OED considered in this book. This is mainly based in optimizing convex objective functions of the covariance matrix of the estimates of the parameters, either in regression, ANOVA, or the mixtures of both types of explanatory variables (Analysis of the Covariance, ANCOVA). In the latter case a numerical explanatory variable is frequently called *covariate*. Of course, OED is model-oriented, but not determined by its structure as it happens with the classical DOE for ANOVA.

Appendix D
Response Surface Analysis Through an Illustrative Example

The ingredients of the problem here are several numerical explanatory variables, x, and a response variable, y, to be optimized (maximized), in function of the values of x. There is the chance to observe y for chosen values of x. This is like trying to climb a mountain with the eyes blindfolded. First, we check whether we are near the top of the mountain trying movements in different directions. If there is a feeling of going down, we must be in the top, meaning that a quadratic model fits significantly better than a linear model. If this is not the case the effort made in each movement will be proportional to the gradient. Fitting a linear model will give the gradient of maximum slope. Then we will try that direction until a feeling of going down appears. Then the process is being repeated until the quadratic model adjusted is significantly better.

A real example will illustrate this procedure (Arévalo-Villena et al., 2011). In the process of wine fermentation there are different variables to be optimized. Specifically, the aim consists in finding conditions for maximizing the enzymatic activity (response variable). It is particularly important to detect the action of a peptide in it. The explanatory variables considered in a first step are reduced to two levels each one (Table D.1). The steps of the whole process are summarized as follows for this example:

1. Identify significant factors using a replicated two-level factorial design 2^5 for the standard levels. In this case two factors were chosen: SHAKING and PEPTIDE.
2. A factorial design 2^2 + 3 central points for these two factors was used.
3. Linear and quadratic fitting were made and a discrimination test between linear and quadratic models was performed.

    - If the linear model is not significantly worse than the quadratic model, then we should search in the direction of the gradient of the plane adjusted until the response decreases.

J. López-Fidalgo, *Optimal Experimental Design*, Lecture Notes in Statistics 226,
https://doi.org/10.1007/978-3-031-35918-7

Table D.1 Two-level explanatory variables

SHAKING	TEMPERATURE	TWEEN	TIME	PEPTIDE
20 rpm (1)	18° C (1)	With (1)	12 hours (1)	With (1)
150 rpm (-1)	28° (-1)	Without (-1)	48 hours (-1)	Without (-1)

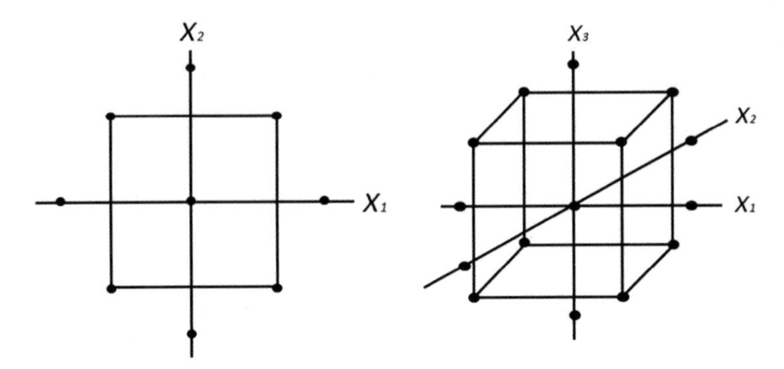

Fig. D.1 Star and composite designs

- If the quadratic model is significantly better, we should use again a composite design with a star design with distance to the center $1 + \alpha$ (α is frequently chosen as $\sqrt{2}$). Figure D.1 shows some examples in two and three dimensions.

4. Canonical analysis of the fitted quadratic model, that is, plotting the contour plot and study the situation. We may have the following situations:
   - If the aspect of the plot is similar to Fig. D.2a, a saddle point is there and we should get out trying in both maximizing directions.
   - Figure D.2b shows an edge and we must search in both directions of it to see whether at some point the surface starts to increase.
   - Figure D.2c shows a parabola letting clear a maximizing direction.
   - Otherwise, Fig. D.2d shows a local maximum is there and we only need to compute it using the fitted polynomial. This is actually the end of the procedure.

   In the example considered the final polynomial fitted was

$$y = -98.78 + 1294\, S + 6.99\, P - 0.0039\, S^2 - 0.1828\, P^2 - 0.00788\, SP,$$

where S is the shacking variable and P is the peptide quantity. Figure D.3 shows the surface. It is easy to find the maximum of this function, which is reached at $S = 150$ rpm and $P = 16$ g/L.

An additional improvement is to include the cost of the peptide in the objective function, which makes sense to avoid too large expenses with this product.

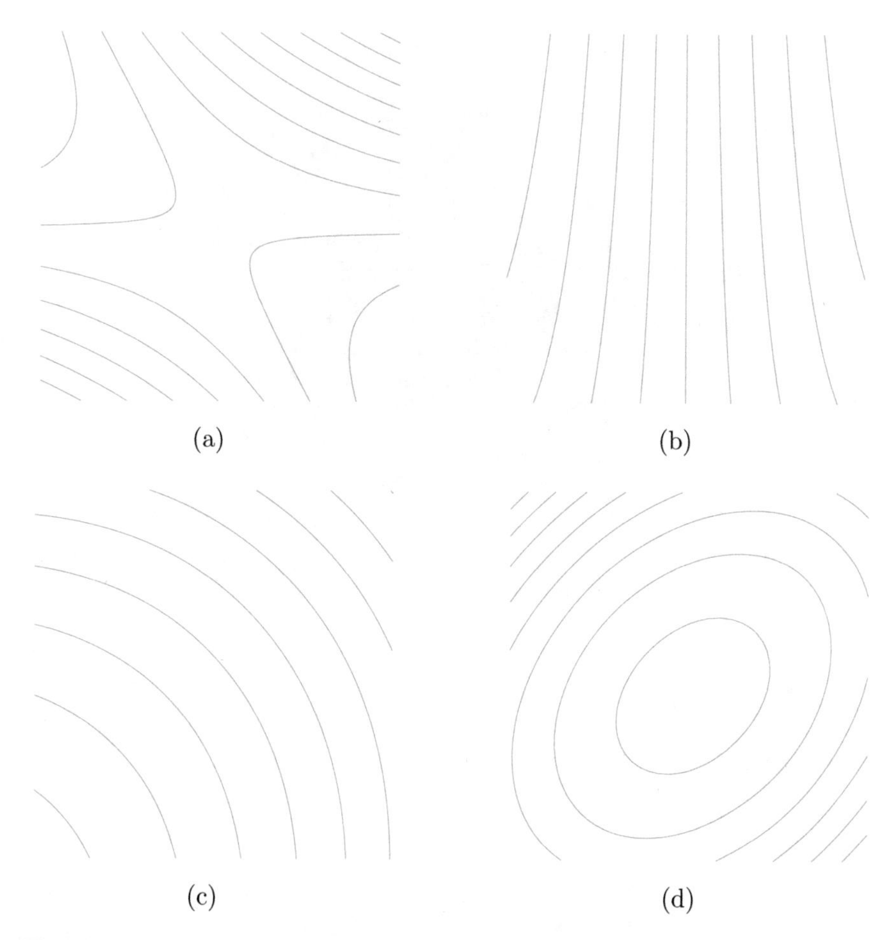

Fig. D.2 Saddle point (**a**), Edge (**b**), Parabola (**c**), Optimal (**d**)

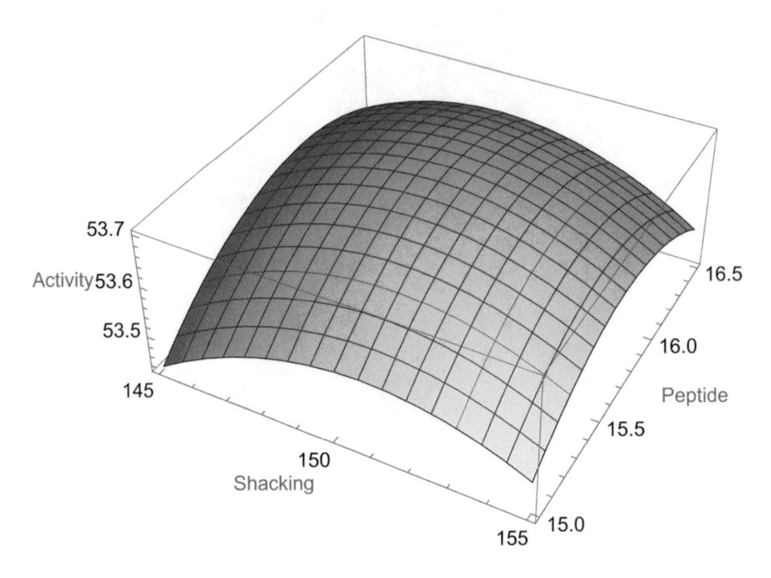

Fig. D.3 Fitted model in the example

Appendix E
Regression and Correlation

The *Pearson linear correlation coefficient* measures the degree of linear relation between two quantitative variables. This coefficient ranges from -1 to 1 being 0 no correlation at all, -1 if one variable is inversely proportional to the other, and 1 if there is direct proportionality. The typical tests for checking whether there is relationship or not are based on the normality of the variables. Moreover, this coefficient might not detect nonlinear relationships (Fig. E.1). For these reasons other coefficients derived from it can be more adequate. The so-called *Spearman coefficient* is the Pearson coefficient of the ranks, that is, the ordering numbers, of the two variables. This means it can be used even for ordinal variables and the tests used now are not based on normality. Additionally, this coefficient detects nonlinear monotonic relationships.

A statistically significant coefficient does not imply causality. It has to be analyzed carefully. Thus, the problem of spurious relationships where the statistical relation is caused by a third variable can be taken over using *partial correlation*, which measures the correlation between two variables eliminating the influence of third variables.

To interpret these coefficients it is important to follow the procedure in two steps. First, check with the appropriate test whether it is significant or no. If it is significant then use the magnitude of the coefficient. There is a number of classifications of this quantity, all of them conventional and arbitrary. Typically, the absolute value of the coefficient over 0.6 or 0.7 is considered "Strong," while under 0.3 is considered "Weak." Otherwise, there is a "Moderate" relationship.

Thus, if there is significant correlation (linear or not) between two variables, a *regression* model gives the mathematical equation of the relationship. Typical examples are

- Linear:
  - Simple: $y = \alpha_0 + \alpha_1 x + \varepsilon$.
  - Multiple: $y = \alpha_0 + \alpha_1 x_1 + \alpha_2 x_2 + \alpha_3 x_3 + \varepsilon$.

J. López-Fidalgo, *Optimal Experimental Design*, Lecture Notes in Statistics 226,
https://doi.org/10.1007/978-3-031-35918-7

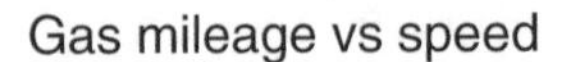

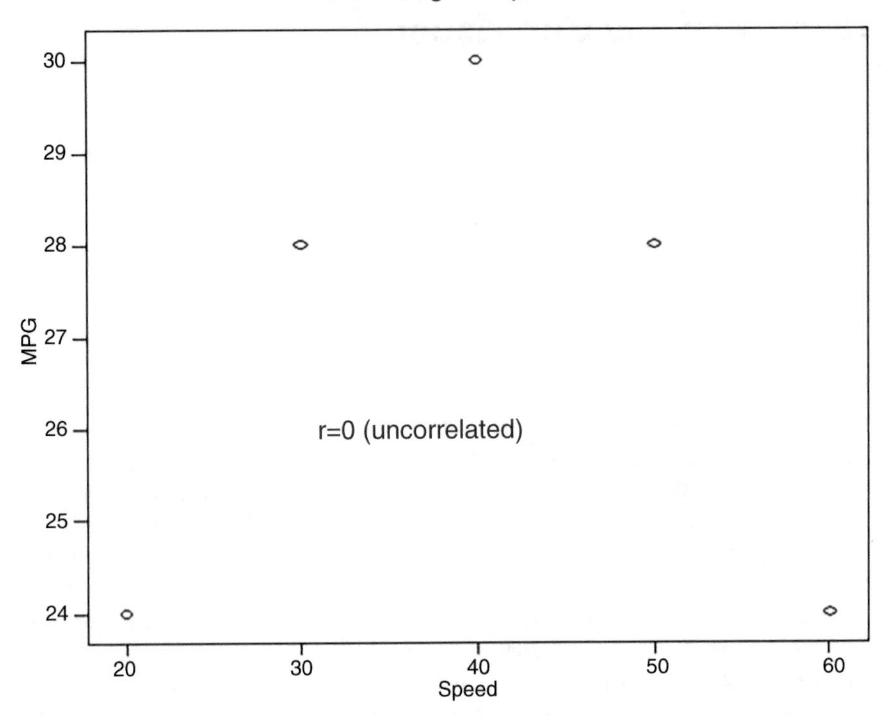

Fig. E.1 Nonlinear correlation relating consumption of gasoline versus the speed of a car

Stepwise regression can be performed here to select appropriate variables to be in the model. The criteria for selecting variables are based on p-values, but also in other indices, such as leverage, to avoid two or more redundant variables live together in the model.

- Nonlinear:
  - In the variables (still called linear model): $y = \alpha_0 + \alpha_1 x^2 + \varepsilon$.
  - In the parameters (nonlinear model): $y = \alpha_0 e^{-\alpha_1 x} + \varepsilon$.
  - Generalized linear models (logistic regression):

$$P(\text{"group 1"}) = P(y = 1) = F(\alpha_0 + \alpha_1 x).$$

Appendix F
Probability Measure Theory

F.1 Measure

Let χ be a sample space. A σ*-algebra* or σ*-field*, $\mathcal{B}$, is a collection of subsets of χ such that

1. $\chi \in \mathcal{B}$.
2. It is closed under complement: If $A \in \mathcal{B}$ then $A^c \in \mathcal{B}$, where A^c is the complement of A.
3. It is closed under countable unions: For all countable collections $\{A_i\}_{i=1}^{\infty}$ of pairwise disjoint sets in $\mathcal{B}$, then $\cup_i A_i \in \mathcal{B}$.

The pair $(\chi, \mathcal{B})$ is called a *measurable space*.

A *measure* on $(\chi, \mathcal{B})$ is a function μ from $\mathcal{B}$ to the extended real number line satisfying the following properties:

1. Nonnegativity: For all $A \in \mathcal{B}$ then $\mu(A) \geq 0$.
2. Null empty set: $\mu(\emptyset) = 0$.
3. Countable additivity (or σ-additivity): For all countable collections $\{A_i\}_{i=1}^{\infty}$ of pairwise disjoint sets in $\mathcal{B}$, then $\mu\left(\bigcup_{i=1}^{\infty} A_i\right) = \sum_{i=1}^{\infty} \mu(A_i)$.

The triple $(\chi, \mathcal{B}, \mu)$ is called a *measure space*.

A *Borel set* is any set in a topological space that can be formed of open sets through the operations of countable union, countable intersection, and relative complement. It is straightforward that the set of all Borel sets is a σ*-algebra*. In particular, the Borel σ-algebra in $\chi \subset \mathbb{R}^p$ will be the collection of all the intersections with χ of all the sets of $\mathbb{R}^p$ formed from open sets through the operations of countable union, countable intersection, and relative complement. We will consider this σ*-algebra* from now on. It is well-known Cartesian products of intervals of the type (x, ∞), $x \in \mathbb{R}$ are generators of the Borel σ-algebra.

A measure, μ, is *discrete* if there exist sequences of real numbers $\{x_i\}_i$ and $\{p_i\}_i$ with $p_i > 0$ and such that $\mu(A) = \sum_{x_i \in A} p_i$. Then μ is the only measure satisfying

J. López-Fidalgo, *Optimal Experimental Design*, Lecture Notes in Statistics 226,
https://doi.org/10.1007/978-3-031-35918-7

that $\mu(\{x_i\}) = p_i$ and $\mu(A) = 0$ if $A \cup \{x_i\}_i = \emptyset$. The points $\{x_i\}_i$ are the atoms of the measure. A measure, μ, is said *finite* if $\mu(\chi) < \infty$.

A *semi-algebra* is a collection of subsets of χ such that

1. It is closed under intersections: If A and B are in the semi-algebra, then $A \cap B$ is in the semi-algebra.
2. If A_1 and A_2 are in the semi-algebra, then there exist $B_1, \dots B_k$ in the semi-algebra such that $A_1 - A_2 = \cap_{i=1}^{k} B_i$.

The *limit superior* and the *limit inferior* of a sequence $\{A_k\}_{k=1}^{\infty}$ are defined as

1. $\overline{\text{limsup}} A_k = \cap_{n=1}^{k} \cup_{k=n}^{\infty} A_i$.
2. $\underline{\text{liminf}} A_k = \cup_{n=1}^{k} \cap_{k=n}^{\infty} A_i$.

In what follows some well-known results in measure theory are provided that will be used later.

Theorem F.1 (Continuity of Measures) *Let μ be a finite measure and let $\{A_n\}_{n\in\mathbb{N}}$ be a sequence of sets of the σ-algebra. Then*

(i) $\mu(\liminf A_n) \leq \liminf \mu(A_n) \leq \limsup \mu(A_n)$.
(ii) If $\{A_n\}_{n\in\mathbb{N}}$ converges, then

$$\mu(\lim_{n\to\infty} A_n) = \lim_{n\to\infty} \mu(A_n).$$

Theorem F.2 (Extension of Measures) *Let $\mu : \mathcal{A} \to \mathbb{R}$ be a measure defined on a semi-algebra $\mathcal{A}$, that is, it is closed for finite intersections and the complement of any set is in $\mathcal{A}$. Then μ can be extended to the σ-algebra $\sigma(\mathcal{A})$ generated by $\mathcal{A}$.*

F.2 Lebesgue Measure and Integration

The *Lebesgue measure* is the traditional measure of the length of an interval in $\mathbb{R}$, that is, $\lambda((a, b)) = \lambda([a, b]) = b - a,\ a, b \in \mathbb{R}$; or likewise the area of a rectangle in $\mathbb{R}^2$. For any other subset of $\mathbb{R}$

$$\lambda(A) = \inf \left\{ \sum_i \lambda(I_i) \mid \{I_i\} \text{ is a sequence of intervals such that } A \subseteq \cup_i I_i \right\}.$$

This definition is consistent just for subsets in the so-called *Lebesgue σ-algebra*. These subsets are called measurable. A set $A \subset \mathbb{R}$ is in that σ-algebra if it satisfies the "Caratheodory criterion" for any $C \subset \mathbb{R}$,

$$\lambda(A) = \lambda(C \cap A) + \lambda(C^c \cap A).$$

The Lebesgue measure generates the traditional integration definition, which generalizes the Riemman integration. Let us define it in progressive steps.

A function $f : \chi \longrightarrow \mathbb{R}$ is said *measurable* if $\{x \mid f(x) > t\} = f^{-1}((t, \infty)) \in \mathcal{B}$ for any $t \in \mathbb{R}$. An *indicator function* of a set $A \in \mathcal{B}$ is defined as

$$\mathbb{1}_A(x) = \begin{cases} 1 \text{ if } x \in A \\ 0 \text{ if } x \notin A. \end{cases}$$

The integral of an indicator is defined as

$$\int \mathbb{1}_A(x) d\lambda = \lambda(A).$$

A *simple function* is defined as a countable linear combination of indicators, $S = \sum_i a_i \mathbb{1}_{A_i}$, and its integral is defined as

$$\int S d\lambda = \sum_i a_i \lambda(A_i).$$

If $B \in \mathcal{B}$ then the defined integral of S at B is

$$\int_B S d\lambda = \int \mathbb{1}_B S d\lambda = \sum_i a_i \lambda(A_i \cap B).$$

If $f \geq 0$ then the integral is defined as

$$\int_\chi f d\lambda = \sup \left\{ \int_\chi S d\lambda \mid 0 \leq S \leq f, \ S \text{ simple function} \right\}.$$

Finally, the generalization for any f comes from the decomposition $f = f^+ - f^-$,

$$\int_\chi f d\lambda = \int_\chi f^+ d\lambda - \int_\chi f^- d\lambda,$$

where

$$f^+(x) = \begin{cases} f(x) \text{ if } f(x) > 0, \\ 0 \quad \text{if } f(x) \leq 0, \end{cases} \qquad f^-(x) = \begin{cases} -f(x) \text{ if } f(x) < 0, \\ 0 \quad \text{if } f(x) \geq 0. \end{cases}$$

The function f is said *integrable* if $\int_\chi |f| d\lambda < \infty$, that is, $f \in L^1$.

F.3 Integration with Respect to a Measure

Let us generalize the Lebesgue integration to any measure space. If $(\chi, \mathcal{B}, \mu)$ is a measure space and $(\mathbb{R}, \mathcal{B}_{\mathbb{R}})$ is the Borel measurable space, a function $f : \chi \longrightarrow \mathbb{R}$ is said *measurable* if $\{x \in \chi \mid f(x) \in B\} \in \mathcal{B}$ for any $B \in \mathcal{B}_{\mathbb{R}}$. Likewise, previous section, a *simple function*, also called *step function*, on a measured space is a measurable function which takes only finitely many values,

$$S = \sum_i a_i \mathbb{1}_{A_i},\ x_i \in \chi,\ a_i = S(x_i) \in \mathbb{R},$$

where $A_i = \{x \in \chi \mid S(x) = a_i\} \in \mathcal{B}$ are disjoint subsets.

This expression is clearly unique, and $S > 0$ if and only if $a_i > 0$ for all i. The set of step functions on χ, denoted by $\mathcal{S}(\chi)$, is closed by product and sum,

$$\mathbb{1}_A \mathbb{1}_B = \mathbb{1}_{A \cap B},\ \mathbb{1}_A + \mathbb{1}_B = \mathbb{1}_{A \cap B} + \mathbb{1}_{A \cup B} = 2 \cdot \mathbb{1}_{A \cap B} + \mathbb{1}_{A \cup B - A \cap B},$$

which is a simple function because $A \cap B$ and $A \cup B - A \cap B$ are disjoint sets.

We now define the integral of a simple function, following Lebesgue's procedure,

$$\int S d\mu \equiv \int S(x)\mu(dx) = \sum_i a_i \mu(A_i).$$

If $A \in \mathcal{B}$ the integral of S on A is defined as

$$\int_A S d\mu = \sum_i a_i \mu(A_i \cap A).$$

The extension to general functions can be made likewise the Lebesgue integration. We would need some results for applying Caratheodory theorem to the theory of approximate experimental designs.

Theorem F.3 (Dominated Convergence) *Let $\{f_i\}_i$ be a nonincreasing sequence of nonnegative measurable functions with point-wise limit f. Let g be an integrable function such that $|f_i| < g$ for any i. Then f is integrable and*

$$\lim_{i \to \infty} \int f_i d\mu = \int f d\mu.$$

Theorem F.4 *Let f be a measurable function, then there exists a sequence of simple functions $\{S_i\}_i$ such that*

1. *$S_i(x) \le S_{i+1}(x)$ for any x and i.*
2. *$S_i(x) \le f(x)$ for any x.*
3. *$f(x) = \lim_{i \to \infty} S_i(x)$ for any x.*

4. *Convergence is uniform in each set* $\{f \leq M\}$, $M > 0$ *(in particular in* χ *if* f *is bounded).*

Corollary F.1 *If* f *is integrable, then* $\{S_i\}$ *satisfies the dominated convergence and then*

$$\int f d\mu = \lim_{i \to \infty} \int S_i d\mu = \lim_{i \to \infty} \sum_j a_{ij} \mu(A_{ij}),$$

where $S_i = \sum_j a_{ij} \mu(A_{ij})$.

F.4 Probability Measure

A *probability measure*, η, is a measure on the Borel σ-algebra in $\chi \subset \mathbb{R}^p$ such that $\eta(\chi) = 1$. The triplet $(\chi, \mathcal{B}, \eta)$ is called *probability measure space*. Then

$$\eta(A) = \int_A \eta(dx).$$

A *random variable* is a function $X : \chi \to \mathbb{R}$ such that for any set, A, of the Borel σ-algebra on $\mathbb{R}$ then $X^{-1}(A)$ is in the Borel σ-algebra on χ. A probability measure η is associated to it in such a way

$$\eta(X \in A) = \int_A \eta(dx).$$

Since the Borel σ-algebra on $\mathbb{R}$ can be generated by intervals, then the so-called *cumulative distribution function* (cdf) determines the probability measure,

$$F(x) = \eta(X \leq x) = \int_{-\infty}^{x} \eta(dx) = \int_{-\infty}^{x} dF = .$$

A *discrete probability measure*, η, is a discrete measure with atoms $\{x_i\}_i$ and positive weights such that $\sum_i p_i = 1$. The cdf is then like a ladder with jumps at the atoms. A *continuous random variable* is a random variable with continuous cdf. An *absolutely continuous random variable* is a random variable such that there exists a *probability density function* (pdf), $f : \chi \to \mathbb{R}$ such that

$$F(x) = \int_{-\infty}^{z} f(z) dz, \; x \in \mathbb{R}.$$

Any *absolutely continuous random variable* is also continuous, but not the opposite. In a similar way a *mass probability function* can be defined for a discrete probability as $f(x) = \eta(\{x\})$, $x \in \mathbb{R}$ and we still call it in this book the pdf. For a continuous random variable $\eta(\{x\}) = 0\, x \in \mathbb{R}$.

In OED an approximate design has been defined as any probability measure on $(\chi, \mathcal{B}, \eta)$. Then nice results can be used either to check whether a design is optimal or to build algorithms to compute them. Since just a discrete design with finite support can be carried out in practice, we have claimed Caratheodory's theorem to prove that there is always a representative of this type for any FIM. This is true but a formality has to be proved before the reasoning made in Sect. 2.3. Actually, in Sect. 2.3 we only proved that any FIM associated to a discrete probability has a representative probability measure with finite support with a bounded number of points in it.

The following theorems will be needed to prove this rigorously.

Theorem F.5 (Decomposition of Measures) *Let F be a proper cdf, that is, associated to a random variable, can be decomposed as a convex combination*

$$F(x) = \lambda F_c(x) + (1 - \lambda) F_d(x),$$

where F_d is a proper cdf of a discrete random variable and F_c is a proper continuous cdf without atoms, that is, $\mu_c(\{x\}) = 0,\ x \in \chi$.

Theorem F.6 (Helly Bray) *Let F_n be a sequence of cdf converging completely to F, that is, convergence almost sure (a.s.) under independence of the random variables of the sequence. Let $f : \mathbb{R} \to \mathbb{R}$ be a continuous and bounded function. Then*

$$\lim_{n\to\infty} \int f dF_n = \int f dF.$$

We are now in situation of proving that any finite measure is the limit of a sequence of discrete measures.

Theorem F.7 *Let $\mu : \mathcal{B} \longrightarrow \mathbb{R}$ be a finite probability measure. Then, there exists a sequence of discrete measures $\{\mu_n\}_n$ such that*

(i) $\lim_{n\to\infty} \mu_n = \mu$.
(ii) For any continuous and bounded function $f : \chi \longrightarrow \mathbb{R}$,

$$\lim_{n\to\infty} \int f d\mu_n = \int f d\mu.$$

Remark F.1 This result is then valid for probability measures, but not for the Lebesgue measure. Additionally, this is not valid for any measurable function f, but just for a continuous and bounded function.

Proof Let μ be a finite probability measure on $\mathbb{R}$. The decomposition theorem in measure theory allows splitting it within the discrete and the continuous part, μ_c, that is, without atoms, $\mu_c(\{x\}) = 0$ for any $x \in \chi$. Thus, it is enough to concentrate in this second part assuming without loss of generality that μ is continuous. Again, without loss of generality we can consider $\chi = [0, 1]$.

For any integer n let S_n be the set of dyadic rational numbers in [0, 1],

$$S_n = \left\{ \frac{k}{2^n} \mid k = 1, \ldots, 2^n \right\}.$$

Let $A_{k,n} = \left[\frac{k-1}{2^n}, \frac{k}{2^n}\right)$ defining a partition of [0, 1] and $x_{k,n} = \frac{k-1}{2^n} \in A_{k,n}$. Finally, let μ_n be a discrete measure with atoms $x_{k,n}$, $k = 1, \ldots, 2^n$, and weights $p_{k,n} = \mu(A_{k,n})$, that is,

$$\mu_n = \sum_{k=1}^{2^n} p_{k,n} \delta_{x_{k,n}}.$$

Then

$$\mu_n([0, 1]) = \sum_{k=1}^{2^n} p_{k,n} = \sum_{k=1}^{2^n} \mu(A_{k,n}) = \mu\left(\cup_{k=1}^{2^n} A_{k,n}\right) = \mu([0, 1)) = \mu([0, 1]).$$

For any $x \in \chi = [0, 1]$, let $k_x = [x2^n]$ be the greatest integer satisfying $k/2^n \leq x$. Then

$$[0, x] = C_n \cup \bigcup_{k \mid k/2^n \leq x} A_{k,n},$$

where $C_n = [K_x/2^n, x]$. Then

$$\begin{aligned}
\mu([0, x]) &= \mu(C_n) + \sum_{k}^{k_x} \mu(A_{k,n}) = \mu(C_n) + \sum_{k}^{k_x} p_{k,n} \\
&= \mu(C_n) + \sum_{x_{k,n} \in [0,1]} p_{k,n} \\
&= \mu(C_n) + \mu_n([0, x]).
\end{aligned}$$

But

$$\lim_{n \to \infty} C_n = \lim_{n \to \infty} \left[\frac{[x2^n]}{2^n}, x\right] = \{x\}.$$

Using the second part of the Theorem F.1 of continuity of measures,

$$\lim_{n\to\infty}[\mu([0,x])-\mu_n([0,x])]=\lim_{n\to\infty}\mu(C_n)=\mu(\lim_{n\to\infty}C_n)=\mu(\{x\})=0.$$

Thus,

$$\lim_{n\to\infty}\mu_n([0,x])=\mu([0,x]).$$

The class of intervals $\{[0,x)\}_{x\in[0,1]}$ generates $\mathcal{B}$. Using the theorem of measures extension F.2, then the limit can be extended to the whole Borel σ-algebra. The theorem of Helly Bray F.6 gives the final result.

If $\chi=\mathbb{R}^+$ the proof can be generalized defining

$$x_{k,n}=\frac{k}{2^n},$$
$$A_{k,n}=[x_{k-1,n},x_{k,n}),\ k=1,\ldots,n2^n,$$
$$A_{n2^n+1,n}=[n,\infty).$$

The intervals $A_{k,n}=[x_{k-1,n},x_{k,n}),\ k=1,\ldots,n2^n+1$ define a partition in $\mathbb{R}^+$. Let μ_n be the discrete measure with atoms $x_{k,n}$ and weights $p_{k,n}=\mu(A_{k,n})$, that is,

$$\mu_n=\sum_{k=1}^{n2^n}p_{k,n}\delta_{x_{k,n}}.$$

Then

$$\mu(\mathbb{R}^+)=\mu_n(\mathbb{R}^+)=\sum_{k=1}^{n2^n}p_{k,n}.$$

If $x\in\mathbb{R}^+$ and $x<n$, then $\mu([0,x])-\mu_n([0,x])=\mu(C)$, where

$$C=C_n=\left[\frac{[x2^n]}{2^n},x\right]\downarrow\{x\}.$$

The second part of the theorem of continuity F.1 of measures gives

$$\lim_{n\to\infty}[\mu([0,x])-\mu_n([0,x])]=\lim_{n\to\infty}\mu(C_n)=\mu(\lim_{n\to\infty}C_n)=\mu(x)=0,$$

and the corresponding cdfs satisfy

$$\lim_{n\to\infty} F_n(x) = F(x),\ x \in \chi,$$

and the theorem of Helly Bray gives the final result for $\chi = \mathbb{R}^+$.

The more general case $\chi = \mathbb{R}$ reduces to the sum of two measures, one on $\mathbb{R}^+$ and one on $\mathbb{R}^-$. □

The next theorem proves that $\mathcal{M}$ is compact if χ is compact and f continuous.

Theorem F.8 *If χ is a compact set on $\mathbb{R}^p$ and f continuous on χ, then the convex hull of all one-point information matrices, $f(x)f^T(x)$, is compact.*

Proof The convex hull of a bounded set on a Euclidean space is compact since it is bounded and closed by definition. Thus, we only need to prove that the set of all one-point information matrices, $f(x)f^T(x)$, is bounded. But the continuous function assigning $x \in \chi$ to $f(x)f^T(x)$ maps the compact set χ into another compact, and so bounded, set $\{f(x)f^T(x) \mid x \in \chi\}$. □

Remark F.2 Let ζ be an approximate design, that is, any probability measure on a design space χ, compact set of a Euclidean space, with the usual Borel σ-algebra. Caratheodory's theorem can be applied to the convex hull of the information matrices associated to designs with mass 1 at just one point. The convex hull is then the set of all finite convex combinations of these matrices. Thus, it can only be applied to discrete designs. The question is whether the information matrix associated to any design is also in this convex hull. If so, the theorem applies to any design. Previous theorem states that for any probability measure, ζ, there exists a sequence of discrete designs, $\{\zeta_n\}$, converging to it. Then ii) guarantees for the information matrices that

$$M(\zeta) = \int f(x)f^T(x)d\zeta = \lim_{n\to\infty} \sum f(x)f^T(x)\zeta_n(\{x\}) = \lim_{n\to\infty} \sum M(\zeta_n),$$

where $f(x)$ are the usual regressors of the model. This means any information matrix is in the interior or in the boundary of the convex hull. Since $\mathcal{M}$ is compact and so closed, then the FIM $M(\zeta)$ for any probability measure ζ is in the convex hull, which actually coincides with $\mathcal{M}$.

F.5 Convergences of Random Variables

A random variable is a function on the sample space with a probability distribution. Thus, given a sequence of r.v.'s $\{X_n\}$, there are different possible definitions of convergence to another r.v. X,

In distribution (in law): $X_n \overset{\mathcal{L}}{\to} X$ as $n \to \infty$ if the sequence of cdfs tends to the cdf of X, $\lim_{n\to\infty} F_n(x) = F(x)$ for every x where F is continuous.

In probability: $X_n \xrightarrow{P} X$ as $n \to \infty$ if $\lim_{n\to\infty} P(|X_n - X| > \varepsilon) = 0$ for every $\varepsilon > 0$.

Almost sure (a.s.): $X_n \xrightarrow{a.s.} X$ as $n \to \infty$ if $P(\lim_{n\to\infty} X_n = X) = 1$.

In mean: $X_n \xrightarrow{L^p} X$ as $n \to \infty$ if $\lim_{n\to\infty} E(|X_n - X|^p) = 0$, $p \geq 1$.

Almost sure convergence implies convergence in probability. Convergence in mean of order p implies converges in mean of order $q < p$. Convergence in mean implies convergence in probability. Convergence in probability implies convergence in distribution.

Let a sequence of estimators, $\hat{\theta}_n$, of a parameter θ for different values of the sample size n. It is said *consistent* if $\hat{\theta}_n \xrightarrow{P} \theta$. The proof of this property is frequently based on the law of large numbers. There are two different versions of these law, the strong and the weak laws of large numbers,

Weak: $\bar{X}_n \xrightarrow{P} \mu$. This is satisfied for any sequence of r.v.'s $\{X_n\}$ independent and identically distributed (iid) with finite expectation $E(X_n) = \mu$ and finite variance. This is still valid if the variances are different for each n, but bounded. If $E(X_n) = \mu_n$ this law can be applied to the sequence $\{X_n - \mu_n\}$ with mean zero.

Strong: $\bar{X}_n \xrightarrow{a.e.} \mu$. This law needs more hypotheses. For instance, the Kolmogorov's strong law states that if $\sum_{n=1}^{\infty} \frac{1}{n^2} \mathrm{Var}(X_n) < \infty$ then $\bar{X}_n - \mathrm{E}(\bar{X}_n) \xrightarrow{a.e.} 0$.

Appendix G
Convex Theory

Some properties of convex functions and convex sets will be considered here, mainly since this has applications to convex minimization. Let V be a linear space. A *convex set* is a set $C \subseteq V$ such that for any $x, z \in C$ and $\lambda \in [0, 1]$, then $\lambda x + (1-\lambda)z \in C$. Let $S \subseteq V$, the convex hull of S is defined as $\text{Hull}(S) = \bigcup_{S \subseteq C convex} C$. It may be said that Hull(S) is the minimum convex set containing C.

Theorem G.1 *Some properties of a convex set are as follows:*

(i) Closure and interior of a convex set are convex.
(ii) Intersection of convex sets is convex.
(iii) Image and inverse image of a convex under an affine map is convex.
(iv) Cartesian product of convex sets is convex.
(v) Product by a scalar, λC, and sums, $C_1 + C_2$, of convex sets are convex.
(vi) If S is compact then Hull(S) is compact.

Simple proofs of these properties can be found in Lange (2013). The reader is encouraged to prove them since they are quite straightforward using the definition.

An important property with application to optimization is the so-called *separation hyperplane* property. Metric spaces have to be defined for this adding a distance to a set, such as our linear space V. A *distance function* on V is a function $d : V \times V \to \mathbb{R}$, that satisfies the following conditions:

1. $d(x, z) \geq 0$, and $d(x, z) = 0$ if and only if $x = z$.
2. It is symmetric: $d(x, z) = d(z, x)$.
3. It satisfies the triangular inequality: $d(x, z) \leq d(x, u) + d(u, z)$.

Such a distance function is known as a metric. Together with V, it makes up a *metric space*. There are some properties whose proofs can be found, for example, in Lange (2013).

J. López-Fidalgo, *Optimal Experimental Design*, Lecture Notes in Statistics 226,
https://doi.org/10.1007/978-3-031-35918-7

Theorem G.2

1. *Let $C \subseteq V$ be a convex set and $x \in V$. Then there exists at most one $z \in C$ such that $d(x, z) = d(x, C)$, where d is a distance on V. If C is closed then there is just one.*
2. *Separation hyperplane theorem: Let C be a convex set and $x \notin C$. Then there exists a unit vector $s \in V$ and $c \in \mathbb{R}$ such that $s^T x \geq c \geq s^T z$ for any $z \in C$. Moreover, if $x \in \partial C$ then there is a unit vector $v \in V$ such that $v^T x \geq v^T z$ for any $z \in C$.*
3. *As a corollary C is the intersection of closed hyperspaces containing it.*
4. *Carathéodory theorem: Let S be a nonempty set of $\mathbb{R}^n$ and $x \in S$. There exists a convex combination of at most $n + 1$ points of S such that $x = \sum_{i=1}^{n+1} \alpha_i x_i$.*

A *convex function* is any extended real-valued function $\phi : V \to \mathbb{R} \cup \{\pm\infty\}$ which satisfies *Jensen's inequality*, that is, for any $x, z \in V$ and any $\lambda \in [0, 1]$, then

$$\phi(\lambda x + (1 - \lambda)z) \leq \lambda\phi(x) + (1 - \lambda)\phi(z).$$

Equivalently, a convex function is any (extended) real-valued function such that its *epigraph*

$$\{(x, u) \in V \times \mathbb{R} \mid \phi(x) \leq u\}$$

is a convex set.

It is *strictly convex* if for any $x \neq z$,

$$\phi(\lambda x + (1 - \lambda)z) < \lambda\phi(x) + (1 - \lambda)\phi(z).$$

These are some properties of convex functions:

Theorem G.3

1. *The definition applies for any convex combination.*
2. *Norms are convex functions by the triangular inequality,*

$$||\alpha x + (1 - \alpha)z|| \leq ||\alpha x|| + ||(1 - \alpha)z|| = \alpha||x|| + (1 - \alpha)||z||.$$

3. *The distance to a convex set is convex.*
4. *The sets $\{x \in V \mid \phi(x) \leq c\}$ and $\{x \in V \mid \phi(x) < c\}$ are convex for any convex function ϕ and $c \in \mathbb{R}$.*
5. *If ϕ is differentiable on an open convex set $C \subset \mathbb{R}^n$. Then ϕ is convex if and only if $\phi(z) \geq \phi(x) + \phi'(x)(z - x)$ for any $x, z \in C$. Moreover, ϕ is strictly convex if and only if $\phi(z) > \phi(x) + \phi'(x)(z - x)$ for any $x \neq z$.*
6. *If ϕ is twice differentiable and ϕ'' is positive semidefinite for every x, then ϕ is convex.*
7. *If ϕ is convex and ψ is convex and decreasing, then $\psi \circ \phi$ is convex.*

8. *If* $\{\phi_m\}$ *is a sequence of convex functions, then* $\lim_{m\to\infty} \phi_m(x)$ *is convex if it exists.*

A function ϕ is *log-convex* if $\log \phi$ is convex. It satisfies the following properties:

Theorem G.4

1. *It is convex.*
2. *If* ψ *is convex then* $\psi \circ \phi$ *is log-convex.*
3. *The function* $\phi(Ax + b)$ *is log-convex.*
4. *The functions* ϕ^α *and* $\alpha\phi$ *are log-convex for* $\alpha > 0$.
5. *If* ψ *is log-convex then* $\phi + \psi$, $\max\{\phi, \psi\}$, $\phi \cdot \psi$ *are log-convex.*
6. *If* $\{\phi_m\}$ *is a sequence of log-convex functions, then* $\lim_{m\to\infty} \phi(x)$ *is log-convex if there exists and is positive.*

Corollary G.1

1. *Dordon's function* $\phi(x) = \log\left(\sum_{i=1}^{r} e^{z_i^T x}\right)$ *is convex for any real vectors* z_i, $i = 1, \ldots, r$.
2. *The Gamma function,* $\Gamma(x) = \int_0^\infty t^{x-1} e^{-t} dt$, *is convex.*
3. *The determinant,* $\phi(\Sigma) = \det \Sigma$, *is log-concave in the space of symmetric positive semidefinite matrices.*

Theorem G.5 *If* ϕ *is a convex function on* C *then it is continuous in the interior of* C *and locally Lipschitz at any interior point* x, *that is, there exist* $c \in \mathbb{R}$ *such that* $|\phi(z) - \phi(z')| \leq c||z - z'||$ *far any* z *and* z' *near* x.

Theorem G.6 *If* ϕ *is a convex function on* $C \subset \mathbb{R}^n$ *then* x *is a local minimum if and only if* $\{z \in C \mid \phi(z) = \phi(x)\}$ *is convex. Then it is a global minimum. If* ϕ *is strictly convex then* $\{z \in C \mid \phi(z) = \phi(x)\}$ *reduces to one point.*

Theorem G.7 *If* ϕ *is a convex function on* $C \subset \mathbb{R}^n$ *then* x *is a global minimum if and only if* $\partial\phi(x, v) \geq 0$ *for any* $v \in C$.

The *dual space* of V is the vector space $V^\star$ of all the linear functions, $V \longrightarrow \mathbb{R}$, with the sum of functions and the product of a function by a scalar in it. Notice that for any $x \in V$ an element associated naturally in the dual of V can be defined as $x^{\star\star}(\phi) = \phi(x), \phi \in V^\star$.

A function ϕ is *symmetric* if $\phi(x) = \phi(z)$ whenever the components of z are a permutation of the components of x.

The *Fenchel conjugate* of a convex function ϕ on V is

$$\phi^\star(z) = \sup_{x \in V} \left\{ z^T x - \phi(x) \right\}.$$

Proposition G.1 *These are some useful properties of Fenchel conjugate:*

(i) *The function* $\phi^\star$ *is also convex.*
(ii) *Let* $\phi_0(x) = \phi(x - v)$, *then* $\phi_0^\star(x) = \phi^\star(x) + v^T x$.

(iii) *It is additive,* $(\sum_i \phi_i)^\star = \sum_i \phi_i^\star$ *and multiplicative by scalars* $(\lambda\phi)^\star = \lambda\phi^\star$.
(iv) *Let* ϕ_0 *be a convex function such that* $\phi_0(x) \leq \phi(x)$ *for every* x, *then* $\phi_0^\star(z) \geq \phi^\star(z)$ *for every* z.
(v) *The following inequality holds,* $\phi^\star(z) + \phi(x) \geq z^T x$.
(vi) *Duality is based on this result,* $\phi_{(0)}^\star = -\inf_x \phi(x)$.

The *biconjugate* of a function ϕ is the conjugate of the conjugate, typically written as $\phi^{\star\star}$. The biconjugate is useful for showing when strong or weak duality holds.

Fenchel–Young inequality: For any $x \in V$ then $\phi^{\star\star}(x) \leq \phi(x)$.

Fenchel–Moreau theorem: $\phi = \phi^{\star\star}$ if and only if ϕ is convex and lower semicontinuous (continuous from the left).

There are a number of inequalities on the moments of random variables of much interest in optimization. In what follows some of them are enumerated.

Proposition G.2

1. $|E(XZ)| \leq [E(X)]^{1/2}[E(Z)]^{1/2}$.
2. *Markov inequality: Let* $g \geq 0$ *be a real increasing function, then* $P(X \geq c) \leq \frac{E[g(X)]}{g(c)}$ *for any real number* c *such that* $g(c) > 0$.
3. *Chernoff bound is a particular case of Markov inequality for* X *Gaussian:* $P(X \geq c) \leq e^{-c^2/2}$.
4. *Chebyshev inequality is also a particular case of Markov inequality:* $P(|X - E(X)| \geq c) \leq \frac{var[X]}{c^2}$.
5. *Jensen inequality: If* g *is convex on the domain of* X *then* $|E[g(X)] \geq g[E(X)]$.
6. *Schlömilch inequality: For any r.v.* $X \geq 0$, $[E(X^p)]^{q/p} \leq E(X^q)$, $0 < q < p$ *and* $E(\log X^p) \leq \log E(X^p)$.
7. *Hölder inequality: For any r.v.* X *and* Z, $E(XZ) \leq [E(|X|^p)]^{1/p}[E(|Z|^p)]^{1/p}$, $0 < q < p$ *and* $E(\log X^p) \leq \log E(X^p)$.

A convex minimization (*primal*) problem is one of the form

$$\inf_{x \in C} \phi(x).$$

such that $\phi : C \to \mathbb{R} \cup \{\pm\infty\}$ is a convex function and $C \subset V$ is a convex set.

In optimization theory, the duality principle states that optimization problems may be viewed from either of two perspectives, the primal problem or the dual problem.

Bibliography

Abt, M. (1998). Approximating the mean squared prediction error in linear models under the family of exponentials correlations. *Statistica Sinica, 8*, 511–526.

Amo-Salas, M., López-Fidalgo, J., & Rodríguez-Díaz, J. M. (2010). Optimizing the test power for a radiation retention model. *Pharmaceutical Statistics, 9*, 55–66.

Amo-Salas, M., López-Fidalgo, J., & López-Rios, V. I. (2012). Optimal designs for two nested pharmacokinetic models with correlated observations. *Communications in Statistics-Simulation and Computation, 41*(7, SI), 944–963. 6th St Petersburg Workshop on Simulation, St Petersburg, RUSSIA, JUN 28–JUL 03, 2009.

Amo-Salas, M., López-Fidalgo, J., & Porcu, E. (2013). Optimal designs for some stochastic processes whose covariance is a function of the mean. *TEST, 22*(1), 159–181.

Amo-Salas, M., López-Fidalgo, J., & Pedregal, D. J. (2015). Experimental designs for autoregressive models applied to industrial maintenance. *Reliability Engineering & System Safety, 133*, 87–94.

Arévalo-Villena, M., Fernández-Guerrero, M. M., López-Fidalgo, J., & Briones-Pérez, A. I. (2011). Pectinases yeast production using grape skin as carbon source. *Advances in Bioscience and Biotechnology, 2*(2), 89–96.

Atkinson, A. (1972). Planning experiments to detect inadequate regression models. *Biometrika, 59*, 275–293.

Atkinson, A. (2008). Dt-optimum designs for model discrimination and parameter estimation. *Journal of Statistical Planning and Inference, 1*, 56–64.

Atkinson, A., & Fedorov, V. (1988). The optimum design of experiments in the presence of uncontrolled variability and prior information. In Y. Dodge, V. Fedorov, & H. P. Wynn (Eds.), *Optimal designs and analysis of experiments*. Amsterdam: North Holland.

Atkinson, A. C., & Donev, A. N. (1992). *Optimum Experimental Designs*. New York: Oxford University Press.

Atkinson, A. C., Donev, A., & Tobias, R. (2007a). *Optimum Experimental Designs, with SAS*. Oxford: Oxford University Press.

Atkinson, A. C., & Cox, D. R. (1974). Planning experiments for discriminating between models. *Journal of the Royal Statistical Society Series B: Statistical Methodology, 36*, 321–348.

Atkinson, A. C., & Fedorov, V. (1975a). The design of experiments for discriminating between two rival models. *Biometrika, 62*(1), 57–70.

Atkinson, A. C., & Fedorov, V. (1975b). Optimal design: Experiments for discriminating between several models. *Biometrika, 62*, 289–303.

Atkinson, A. C., Pronzato, L., & Wynn, W. P. (Eds.). (1998). *MODA 5: Advances in Model-oriented data analysis and experimental design* Heidelberg: Springer.

J. López-Fidalgo, *Optimal Experimental Design*, Lecture Notes in Statistics 226,
https://doi.org/10.1007/978-3-031-35918-7

Atkinson, A. C., Bogacka, B., & Zhigljavsky, A. (Eds.). (2001a). *Optimum design 2000. Nonconvex Optimum Applications*, vol. 51. Dordrecht: Kluwer Academic Publishers.

Atkinson, A. C., Hackl, P., & Müller, W. (Eds.). (2001b). *MODA 6: Advances in model-oriented design and analysis*. Heidelberg: Physica Verlag.

Atkinson, A. C., Donev, A. N., & Tobias, R. D. (2007b). *Optimum Experimental Designs, with SAS*. Oxford: Oxford University Press.

Atkinson, A. C., Uciński, D., & Patan, M. (Eds.). (2013). *mODa10: Advances on model-oriented design and analysis*. Heidelberg: Physica Verlag.

Atwood, C. L. (1969). Optimal and efficient designs of experiments. *The Annals of Mathematical Statistics, 40*(5), 1570–1602.

Atwood, C. L. (1976). Convergent design sequences, for sufficiently regular optimality criteria. *The Annals of Statistics, 1*(2), 342–352.

Bailey, R. A. (2008). *Design of Comparative Experiments*. Cambridge: Cambridge University Press.

Bartroff, J. (2011). A new characterization of Elfving's method for high dimensional computation. *Journal of Statistical Planning and Inference, 142*(4), 863–871.

Beckenbach, E. F., & Bellman, R. (1965). *Inequalities*. Berlin: Springer.

Berg, C., Mateu, J., & Porcu, E. (2008). The Dagum family of isotropic correlation functions. *Bernoulli, 14*, 1134–49.

Berger, J. O. (1985). *Statistical Decision Theory and Bayesian Analysis*. New York: Springer.

Berger, M. P. F., & Wong, W. K. (Eds.). (2005). *Applied Optimal Designs*. New York: Wiley.

Berger, M. P. F., & Wong, W. K. (2009). *An Introduction to Optimal Designs for Social and Biomedical Research*. New York: Wiley.

Bernardo, J. M. (1979). Expected information as expected utility. *Annals of Statistics, 7*, 686–690.

Biedermann, S., Dette, H., & Pepelyshev, A. (2007). Optimal discrimination designs for exponential regression models. *Journal of Statistical Planning and Inference, 137*, 2579–2592.

Bischoff, W., & Miller, F. (2006). Optimal designs which are efficient for lack of fit tests. *The Annals of Statistics, 34*, 2015–2025.

Box, G. E. P., & Hunter, W. G. (1965). *IBM Scientific Computing Symposium in Statistics*. Chapter Sequential design of experiments for non-linear models, pp. 111–137. New York: IBM, White Plains.

Box, G. E. P. (1979). Some problems of statistics and everyday life. *Journal of the American Statistical Association, 74*, 1–4.

Braess, D., & Dette, H. (2013). Optimal discriminating designs for several competing regression models. *Annals of Statistics, 1*(2), 897–922.

Brimkulov, U. N., Krug, G. K., & Savanov, V. L. (1986). *Design of experiments in investigating random fields and processes*. Moskow: Nanko (in Russian).

Brooks, R. J. (1972). A decision theory approach to optimal regression designs. *Biometrika, 59*(3), 563–571.

Brooks, R. J. (1976). Optimal regression designs for prediction when prior knowledge is available. *Metrika, 23*, 221–230.

Broudiscou, A., Leardi, R., & Phan-Tan-Luu, R. (1996). Genetic algorithm as a tool for selection of d-optimal design. *Chemometrics and Intelligent Laboratory Systems, 35*, 105–116.

Brown, L. D., Olkin, I., Sacks, J., & Wynn, H. P. (1985). *Jack Carl Kiefer Collected papers III*. New York: Springer.

Campos-Barreiro, S., & López-Fidalgo, J. (2016). KL-Optimal experimental design for discriminating between two growth models applied to a beef farm. *Mathematical Biosciences and Engineering, 13*(1), 67–82.

Carter, M., & van Brunt, B. (2000). *The Lebesgue-Stieltjes integral: A practical introduction*. New York: Springer.

Casero-Alonso, V., & López-Fidalgo, J. (2015). Experimental designs in triangular simultaneous equations models. *Statistical Papers, 56*(2), 273–290.

Celant, G., & Broniatowski, M. (2017). *Interpolation and extrapolation optimal designs 2: Finite dimensional general models*. London: Wiley-ISTE.

Chaloner, K. (1984). Optimal Bayesian experimental designs for linear models. *The Annals of Statistics, 12*, 283–300.

Chaloner, K., & Verdinelli, I. (1995). Bayesian experimental design: A review. *Statistical Science, 10*(3), 273–304.

Chen, P.-Y., Chen, R.-B., & Wong, W. K. (2022). Particle swarm optimization for searching efficient experimental designs: A review. *Wiley Interdisciplinary Reviews-Computational Statistics 14*(5), e1578.

Chen, V. C. P., Tsui, K.-L., Barton, R. R., & Meckesheimer, M. (2009). A review on design, modeling and applications of computer experiments. *IIE Transactions, 38*(4), 273–291.

Chernoff, H. (1953). Locally optimal designs for estimating parameters. *Annals of Mathematical Statistics, 24*, 586–602.

Chernoff, H. (2000). *Sequential Analysis and Optimal Design*. Philadelphia: SIAM Society for Industrial & Applied Mathematics.

Cook, R. D., & Wong, W. K. (1994). On the equivalence of constrained and compound optimal designs. *Journal of the American Statistical Association, 89*, 687–692.

Cook, R.D., & Thibodeau, L. A. (1980). Marginally restricted D-optimal designs. *Journal of the American Statistical Association, 75*(370), 366–371.

Cox, D. R. (1962). Further results on tests of separate families of hypotheses. *Journal of the Royal Statistical Society, Series B, 24*(2), 406–424.

Cressie, N. (1993). *Statistics for spatial data*. New York: Wiley.

DasGupta, A. (2007). Bayesian experimental design. In Montesano, A., Daboni, L., & Lines, M., (Eds.). *Encyclopedia of statistical sciences*. Utrecht: Wiley.

Dean, A. M., Morris, M., Stufken, J., & Bingham, D. (2020). *Handbook of design and analysis of experiments*. New York: Chapman and Hall/CRC.

DeGroot, M. H. (1962). Uncertainty information and sequential experiments. *The Annals of Statistics, 33*, 404–419.

DeGroot, M. H. (1986). Concepts of information based on utility. In Montesano, A., Daboni, L., & Lines, M., (Eds.). *Recent developments in the foundations of utility and risk theory*, pp. 265–275. Reidel: Dordrecht, Holland.

Deldossi, L., Osmetti, S. A., & Tommasi, Ch. (2016). PKL-optimality criterion in copula models for efficacy-toxicity response. In J. Kunert, Ch. Müller, & A. C. Atkinson (Eds.). *MODA 11: Advances in model-oriented data analysis*, pp. 79–86. Heidelberg: Physica Verlag.

Dette, H. (1993a). Elfving's theorem for D-optimality. *The Annals of Statistics, 21*, 753–766.

Dette, H. (1993b). A note on Bayesian c- and D-optimal designs in nonlinear regression models. Technical report, Manuscript.

Dette, H. (1997). Designing experiments with respect to "standardized" optimality criteria. *Journal of the Royal Statistical Society, Series B, 59*(1), 97–110.

Dette, H., & Studden, W. J. (1997). *The theory of canonical moments with applications in statistics*. New York: Wiley.

Dette, H., Melas, V. B., & Wong, W. K. (2006). Locally d-optimal designs for exponential regression models. *Statistica Sinica, 16*, 789–803.

Di Buchianico, A., Laüter, H., & Wynn, H. P. (Eds.). (2004). *MODA 7: Advances in Model-Oriented Design and Analysis*. Heidelberg: Physica Verlag.

Dodge, Y., Fedorov, V., & Wynn, H. P. (Eds.). (1988). *First International Conference—Workshop on Optimal Designs and Analysis of Experiments*. Amsterdam: Elsevier science publishers B. V. North Holland.

Dorta-Guerra, R., González-Dávila, E., & Ginebra, J. (2008). Two-level experiments for binary response data. *Computational Statistics and Data Analysis, 53*, 196–208.

Duarte, B. P. M., & Wong, W. K. (2014). Finding Bayesian optimal designs for nonlinear models: A semidefinite programming-based approach. *International Statistical Review, 83*(2), 239–262.

Duarte, B. P. M., Granjo, J. F. O., & Wong, W. K. (2020). Optimal exact designs of experiments via mixed integer nonlinear programming. *Statistics and Computing, 30*(1), 93–112.

Eaton, M. L., Giovagnoli, A., & Sebastiani, P. (1994). A predictive approach to the Bayesian design problem with application to normal regression models. Technical report, Minnesota: University of Minnesota.

El Krunz, S.M., & Studden, W. J. (1991). Bayesian optimal designs for linear regression models. *The Annals of Statistics, 17*, 2183–2208.

Elfving, G. (1952). Optimum allocation in linear regression theory. *Annals of Mathematical Statistics, 23*, 255–262.

Fedorov, V. (1972). *Theory of optimal experiments*. New York: Academic Press.

Fedorov, V. (1989). Optimal design with bounded density: Optimization algorithms of the exchange type. *Journal of Statistical Planning and Inference, 22*, 1–13.

Fedorov, V., & Hackl, P. (1997). *Model-Oriented Design of Experiments*. Lecture Notes in Statistics. New York: Springer.

Fedorov, V., & Leonov, S. (2013). *Optimal Design for Nonlinear Response Models*. New York: CRC Press.

Fedorov, V., & Pázman, A. (1968). Design of physical experiments (statistical methods). *Fortschritte der Physik, 24*, 325–345.

Fehr, J., Heiland, J., Himpe, Ch., & Saak, J. (1990). Best practices for replicability, reproducibility and reusability of computer-based experiments exemplified by model reduction software. *AIMS Mathematics, 1*(3), 261–281.

Filova, L., Trnovska, M., & Harman, R. (2012). Computing maximin efficient experimental designs using the methods of semidefinite programming. *Metrika, 75*(5), 709–719.

Flournoy, N., Rosenberger, W. F., & Wong, W. K., (Eds.). (1998). *New developments and applications in experimental design*. IMS Lecture Notes—Monograph Series, vol. 34. Hayward: Institute of Mathematical Statistics.

Garcet-Rodríguez, S., López-Fidalgo, J., & Martín-Martín, R. (2008). Some complexities in optimal experimental designs introduced by real life problems. *Tatra Mountains Mathematical Publications, 39*, 135–143.

García-Ródenas, R., García-García, J. C., López-Fidalgo, J., Martin-Baos, J. A., & Wong, W. K. (2020). A comparison of general-purpose optimization algorithms for finding optimal approximate experimental designs. *Computational Statistics & Data Analysis, 144*, 106844.

Gibilisco, P., Riccomagno, E., Rogantin, M.-P., & Wynn, H. P. (2009). *Algebraic and Geometric Methods in Statistics*. Cambridge: Cambridge University Press.

Giovanolly, A., Atkinson, A., & Torsney, B., (Eds.). (2010). *MODA 9: Advances in model-oriented design and analysis*. Heidelberg: Physica Verlag.

Gneiting, T. (2002). Nonseparable, stationary covariance functions for space-time data. *Journal of the American Statistical Association, 97*(458), 590–600.

Gneiting, T., & Schlather, M. (2004). Stochastic models that separate fractal dimension and the hurst effect. *SIAM Review, 46*, 269–282.

Goos, P., & Jones, B. (2011). *Optimal Design of Experiments: A Case-Study Approach*. New York: Wiley.

Hackl, P. (1995). Optimal designs for experiments with potentially failing trials. In *MODA 4: Advances in Model-Oriented Data Analysis*, pp. 117–124. Physica Verlag: Heidelberg.

Harman, R. (2008). Equivalence theorem for Schur optimality of experimental designs. *Journal of Statistical Planning and Inference, 138*, 1201–1209.

Harman, R., & Jurik, T. (2008). Computing c-optimal experimental designs using the simplex method of linear programming. *Computational Statistics & Data Analysis, 53*(2), 247–254.

Harman, R., & Stulajter, F. (2010). Optimal prediction designs in finite discrete spectrum linear regression models. *Metrika, 72*(2), 281–294.

Harman, R., Filová, L., & Richtárik, P. (2020). A randomized exchange algorithm for computing optimal approximate designs of experiments. *Journal of the American Statistical Association, 115*(519), 348–361.

Harman, R., Mueller, W. G., & Woods, D. (Eds.). (2019). mODa12: Advances in model-oriented design and analysis. *Statistical Papers 60*(5), 351–354.

Harman, R. (2014). Multiplicative methods for computing d-optimal stratified designs of experiments. *Journal of Statistical Planning and Inference, 146*, 82–94.

Harman, R., & Benkova, E. (2017). Barycentric algorithm for computing d-optimal size- and cost-constrained designs of experiments. *Metrika, 80*(2), 201–225.

Harman, R., & Lacko, V. (2010). On decompositional algorithms for uniform sampling from n-spheres and n-balls. *Journal of Multivariate Analysis, 101*(10), 2297–2304.

Harman, R., & Rosa, S. (2020). On greedy heuristics for computing d-efficient saturated subsets. *Operations Research Letters, 48*(2), 122–129.

Harman, R., Bachrata, A., & Filova, L. (2016). Construction of efficient experimental designs under multiple resource constraints. *Applied Stochastic Models in Business and Industry, 32*(1), 3–17.

Imhof, L., & Wong, W. K. (2000). A graphical method for finding maximin designs. *Biometrics, 56*, 113–117.

Imhof, L., Song, D., & Wong, W. K. (2002). Optimal design of experiments with possibly failing trials. *Statistica Sinica* **12**(4), 1145–1155.

Imhof, L., Song, D., & Wong, W. K. (2004). Optimal design of experiments with anticipated pattern of missing observations. *Journal of Theoretical Biology, 228*(2), 251–260.

Imhof, L., López-Fidalgo, J., & Wong, W. K. (2001). Efficiencies of rounded optimal approximate designs for small samples. *Statistica Neerlandica, 55*(3), 301–318.

Karlin, S., & Studden, W. (1966). Optimal experimental designs. *Annals of Mathematical Statistics, 37*, 783–810.

Kiefer, J. (1959). Optimum experimental designs. *Journal of the Royal Statistical Society: Series B, 21*, 272–319.

Kiefer, J. (1974). General equivalence theory for optimum designs (Approximate theory). *Annals of Statistics, 2*(5), 848–879.

Kiefer, J., & Wolfowitz, J. (1960). The equivalence of two extremum problems. *Canadian Journal of Mathematics, 12*, 363–366.

Kitsos, Ch., & Müller, W. (Eds.). (1995). *MODA 4: Advances in model-oriented data analysis*. Heidelberg: Physica Verlag.

Kitsos, C. P. (2013). *Optimal experimental design for non-linear models*. Springer Briefs in Statistics. Heidelberg: Springer.

Konstantinou, M., Biedermann, S., & Kimber, A. C. (2013a). Optimal designs for two-parameter nonlinear models with application to survival models. *Statistica Sinica, 24*(1), 415–428.

Konstantinou, M., Biedermann, S., & Kimber, A. C. (2013b). Optimal designs for full and partial likelihood information—with application to survival models. *Statistica Sinica* (submitted).

Kunert, J., Müller, C.H., & Atkinson, A. C. (Eds.). (2016). *mODa11: Advances on model-oriented design and analysis*. Physica Verlag: Heidelberg.

Lange, K. (2013). *Optimization*. New York: Springer.

Lanteri, A., Leorato, S., Lopez-Fidalgo, J., & Tommasi, Ch. (2023). Designing to detect heteroscedasticity in a regression model. *Journal of The Royal Statistical Society Series B, 85*(2), 315–326.

Lindley, D. V. (1956). On the measure of information provided by an experiment. *The Annals of Statistics, 27*, 986–1005.

Lindley, D. V., & Smith, A. M. F. (1972). Bayes estimates for the linear model. *Journal of the Royal Statistical Society, 34*, 1–41.

Liski, E. P., Mandal, N. K., Shah, K. R., & Sinha, B.-K. (2002). *Topics in Optimal Design*. New York: Springer.

Liu, X., Yue, R. X., Zhang, Z., & Wong, W. K. (2021). G-optimal designs for hierarchical linear models: an equivalence theorem and a nature-inspired meta-heuristic algorithm. *Soft Computing, 25*(21), 13549–13565.

Liu, X., Yue, R. X., Zhang, Z., & Wong, W. K. (2022). G-optimal designs for hierarchical linear models: an equivalence theorem and a nature-inspired meta-heuristic algorithm (vol 25, pp. 13549, 2021). *Soft Computing, 26*(17), 8947.

Logothetis, N., & Wynn, H. P. (1989). *Quality through design: Experimental design, off-line quality control, and Taguchi's contributions*. Oxford: Oxford University Press.

López-Fidalgo, J., & Garcet-Rodríguez, S.A. (2004). Optimal experimental designs when some independent variables are not subject to control. *Journal of the American Statistical Association, 99*(468), 1190–1199.

López-Fidalgo, J., & Rivas-López, M. J. (2014). Optimal experimental designs for partial likelihood information. *Computational Statistics & Data Analysis, 71*, 859–867.

López-Fidalgo, J., & Rivas-López, M. J. (2007). Mv-optimality standardized through the coefficient of variation. *Journal of Statistical Planning and Inference, 137*, 2680–2007.

López-Fidalgo, J., & Rodríguez-Díaz, J. M. (2004). Elfving's method for m-dimensional models. *METRIKA, 59*(3), 235–244.

López-Fidalgo, J., & Sanchez, G. (2005). Statistical criteria to establish bioassay programs. *Health Physics, 89*(4), 333–338.

López-Fidalgo, J., & Tommasi, Ch. (2018). Optimal experimental design for model selection: A partial review. In E. Gil, E. Gil, J. Gil, & M. A. Gil (Eds.). *Mathematics of the uncertain: A tribute to Pedro Gil*. Studies in Systems Decision and Control, vol. 142, pp. 253–263. Berlin: Springer.

López-Fidalgo, J., & Villarroel, J. (2007). Optimal designs for radiation retention with Poisson correlated response. *Statistics in Medicine, 26*(9), 1999–2016.

López Fidalgo, J., & Wong, W. K. (2002). Design for the Michaelis-Menten model. *Journal of Theoretical Biology, 215*, 1–11.

López-Fidalgo, J., Rodríguez-Díaz, J. M., & Torsney, B. (Eds.). (2007). *MODA 8: Advances in model-oriented design and analysis*. Heidelberg: Physica Verlag.

López-Fidalgo, J., Rodríguez-Díaz, J. M., Sanchez, G., & Santos-Martin, M.T. (2005). Optimal designs for compartmental models with correlated observations. *Journal of Applied Statistics, 32*(10), 1075–1088.

López-Fidalgo, J., Rivas-López, M. J., & Fernandez-Garzon, B. (2007a). A-optimality standardized through the coefficient of variation. *Communications in Statistics-Theory and Methods, 36*(1–4), 781–792.

López-Fidalgo, J., Tommasi, C., & Trandafir, P. C. (2007b). An optimal experimental design criterion for discriminating between non-normal models. *Journal of the Royal Statistical Society Series B-Statistical Methodology, 69*(2), 231–242.

López-Fidalgo, J., Martin-Martin, R., & Stehlik, M. (2008a). Marginally restricted D-optimal designs for correlated observations. *Journal of Applied Statistics, 35*(6), 617–632.

López-Fidalgo, J., Tommasi, Ch., & Trandafir, C. (2008b). Optimal designs for discriminating between some extensions of the Michaelis-Menten model. *Journal of Statistical Planning and Inference, 138*(12), 3797–3804.

López-Fidalgo, J., Rivas-López, M. J., & del Campo, R. (2009). Optimal designs for Cox regression. *Statistica Neerlandica, 63*(2), 135–148.

Mandal, S., & Torsney, B. (2000). Algorithms for the construction of optimizing distributions. *Communications in Statistics - Theory and Methods, 29*, 1219–1231.

Martin-Martin, R., Torsney, B., & López-Fidalgo, J. (2007). Construction of marginally and conditionally restricted designs using multiplicative algorithms. *Computational Statistics & Data Analysis, 51*(12), 5547–5561.

Matérn, B. (1986). *Spatial Variation*. Berlin: Springer.

Melas, V. B. (2006). *Functional approach to optimal experimental design*. New York: Springer.

Moler, J. A., Plo, F., & San Miguel, M. (2006). An adaptive design for clinical trials with non-dichotomous response and prognostic factors. *Statistics and Probability Letters, 76*, 1940–1946.

Müller, C. H. H. (1997). *Robust Planning and Analysis of Experiments*. New York: Springer.

Müller, W., Wynn, H., & Zhigljavsky, A. (Eds.). (1993). *Model-Oriented data analysis*, Heidelberg: Physica Verlag.

Müller, W. G. (2007a). *Collecting spatial data: Optimum design of experiments for random fields*. Heidelberg: Springer.

Müller, W.G. (2007b). *Collecting spatial data: Optimum design of experiments for random fields*, 3rd edn. Heidelberg: Physica-Verlag.

Müller, W. G., & Stehlík, M. (2009). Issues in the optimal design of computer simulation experiments. *Applied Stochastic Models in Business and Industry, 25*, 163–177.

O'Brien, T. (1995). Optimal design and lack of fit in nonlinear regression models. *Statistical Modelling, 104*, 2601–2617.

Pázman, A. (1986). *Foundations of optimum experimental design*. Dordrecht: D. Reidel Publishing Company.

Pázman, A. (2004). *Correlated optimum design with a parametrized covariance function*. Technical report, Wirtschaftsuniversität, Vienna: Department of Statistics and Mathematics.

Pázman, A. (2007). Criteria for optimal design of small-sample experiments with correlated observations. *Kybernetika, 43*(4), 453–462.

Pázman, A. (2010). Information contained in design points of experiments with correlated observations. *Kybernetika, 4*(6), 771–783.

Pázman, A., Hainy, M., & Müller, W. G. (2022). A convex approach to optimum design of experiments with correlated observations. *Electronic Journal of Statistics, 16*, 5659–5691.

Pilz, J. (1993). *Bayesian estimation and experimental design in linear regression models*. New York: Wiley.

Ponce de Leon, A., & Atkinson A. (1992). *Advances in GLM and Statistical Modelling*. chapter The design of experiments to discriminate between two rival generalized linear models, pp. 159–164. Lecture Notes in Statistics. New York: Springer.

Pronzato, L., & Pázman, A. (2013). *Design of Experiments in Nonlinear Models: Asymptotic Normality, Optimality Criteria and Small-Sample Properties*. New York: Springer.

Pronzato, L., & Zhigljavsky, A. A. (2008). *Optimal design and related areas in optimization and statistics*. New York: Springer.

Pukelsheim, F. (1993). *Optimal design of experiments*. New York: Wiley.

Pukelsheim, F., & Rieder, S. (1992). Efficient rounding of approximate designs. *Biometrika, 79*(4), 763–770.

Pukelsheim, F., & Rosenberger, J. L. (1993). Experimental designs for model discrimination. *Journal of the American Statistical Association, 88*(442), 642–649.

Pukelsheim, F., & Torsney, B. (1991). Optimal weights for experimental designs on linearly independent support points. *The Annals of Statistics, 19*(3), 1614–1625.

Rasch, D., & Darius, P. (1995). *Computer Aided Design of Experiments*. Computational Statistics. Heidelberg: Physica-Verlag.

Rasch, D., Pilz, J., & Simecek, P. (2010). *Optimal experimental design with R*. London: Taylor & Francis.

Rivas-López, M. J., López-Fidalgo, J., & del Campo, R. (2014). Optimal experimental designs for accelerated failure time with Type I and random censoring. *Biometrical Journal, 56*(5, SI), 819–837.

Rodríguez-Díaz, J. M., & López-Fidalgo, J. (2003). A bidimensional class of optimality criteria involving phi(p) and characteristic criteria. *Statistics, 37*(4), 325–334.

Rosa, S., & Harman, R. (2022). Computing minimum-volume enclosing ellipsoids for large datasets. *Computational Statistics & Data Analysis, 171*, 107452.

Sacks, J., Welch, W. J., Mitchell, T. J., & Wynn, H. P. (1989). Design and analysis of computer experiments. *Statistical Science, 4*(4), 409–423.

Sagnol, G., & Harman, R. (2015). Computing exact d-optimal designs by mixed integer second-order cone programming. *Annals of Statistics, 43*(5), 2198–2224.

San Martini, A., & Spezzaferri, F. (1984). A predictive model selection criterion. *Journal of the Royal Statistical Society: Series B (Methodological), 46*, 296–303.

Sánchez, G. (2007). Fitting bioassay data and performing uncertainty analysis with BIOKMOD. *Health Physics, 2*(1), 64–72.

Sánchez, G., & Rodríguez-Díaz, J. M. (2007). Optimal design and mathematical model applied to establish bioassay programs. *Radiation Protection Dosimetry, 123*(4), 457–463.

Schwabe, R. (1996). *Optimum designs for multi-factor models*. New York: Springer.

Shah, K. R., & Sinha, B. K. (1989). *Theory of Optimal Design*. Lecture Notes in Statistics. New York: Springer.

Shannon, C. E.: A mathematical theory of communication. *Bell System Technical Journal, 27*, 379–423, 623–656 (1948)

Silvey, S. D. (1980). *Optimal design*. London: Chapman & Hall.

Silvey, S. D., & Titterington, D. M. (1973). A geometric approach to optimal design theory. *Biometrika, 60*(1), 21–32.

Smith, K. (1918). On the standard deviations of adjusted and interpolates values of an observed polynomial functions and its constants and the guidance they give towards a proper choice of the distribution of observations. *Biometrika, 12*, 1–85.

Spezzaferri, F. (1988). Nonsequential designs for model discrimination and parameter estimation. In D. V. Lindley, J. M. Bernardo, M. H. DeGroot, & A. F. M. Smith, (Eds.). *Bayesian Statistics*, pp. 777–783. Oxford: Oxford University Press.

Stacy, E. W. (1962). A generalization of the gamma distribution. *Annals of Mathematical Statistics, 33*(3), 407.

Stokes, Z., Mandal, A., & Wong, W. K. (2020). Using differential evolution to design optimal experiments. *Chemometrics and Intelligent Laboratory Systems, 199*, 103955.

Stone, M. (1959a). Application of a measure of information to the design and comparison of regression experiments. *The Annals of Mathematical Statistics, 3*, 55–70.

Stone, M. (1959b). Discussion of Kiefer. *Journal of the Royal Statistical Society: Series B, 21*, 313–315.

Taguchi, G. (1986). *Introduction to quality engineering*. Tokyo: Asian Productivity Organization.

Tiao, G. C., & Afonja, B. (1976). Some Bayesian considerations of the choice of design for ranking selection and estimation. *Annals of the Institute of Statistical Mathematics, 28*, 167–186.

Tibshirani, R. (1996). Regression shrinkage and selection via the Lasso. *Journal of the Royal Statistical Society Series B-Statistical Methodology, 58*(1), 267–288.

Tommasi, C. (2007). Optimal designs for discriminating among several non-normal models. In J. López-Fidalgo, J. Rodríguez-Díaz, & B. J. M. Torsney (Eds.). *Advances in model-oriented design and analysis mODa 8*, pp. 213–220. Heidelberg: Physica-Verlag.

Tommasi, C. (2009). Optimal designs for both model discrimination and parameter estimation. *Journal of Statistical Planning and Inference, 139*, 4123–4132.

Tommasi, C., & López-Fidalgo, J. (2010). Bayesian optimum designs for discriminating between models with any distribution. *Computational Statistics & Data Analysis, 54*(1), 143–150.

Tommasi, Ch., Martín-Martín, R., & López-Fidalgo J. (2016). Max–min optimal discriminating designs for several statistical models. *Computational Statistics & Data Analysis, 26*(6), 1163–1172.

Torsney, B. (1983). A moment inequality and monotonicity of an algorithm. In K. O. Kortanek, & A. V. Fiacco (Eds.). *Proceedings of the International Symposium on Semi-Infinite Programming and Applications*. Lecture Notes in Economics and Mathematical Systems, vol. 215, pp. 249–260. Austin: University of Texas.

Ucinski, D., & Atkinson, A. C. (2004). Experimental design for time-dependent models with correlated observations. *Studies in Nonlinear Dynamics & Econometrics, 8*(2), 13.

Ucinski, D., & Bogacka, B. (2004). $T-$optimum designs for multiresponse dynamic heteroscedastic models. In *7th International Workshop on Model-Oriented Design and Analysis, MODA7*, pp. 167–174. Berlin: Springer.

Varela, G., Cordovilla, R., Jiménez, M. F., & Novoa, N. (2001). Utility of standardized exercise oximetry to predict cardiopulmonary morbidity after lung resection. *European Journal of Cardio-thoracic Surgery, 19*, 351–354.

Vazquez, A. R., Wong, W. K., & Goos, P. (2023). Constructing two-level q(b)-optimal screening designs using mixed-integer programming and heuristic algorithms. *Statistics and Computing, 33*, 7.

Verdinelli, I., Polson, N., & Singpurwalla, N. (1993). Shannon information and Bayesian design for prediction in accelerated life testing. In R. E. Barlow, C. A. Clarotti, & F. Spizzichino, (Eds.). *Reliability and Decision Making*, pp. 247–256. London: Chapman and Hall.

Wald, A. (1943). On the efficient design of statistical investigations. *Annals of Mathematical Statistics, 14*, 134–140.

Walter, E., & Pronzato, L. (1997). *Identification of parametric models from experimental data.* London: Springer.

Wang, H.-Y., Yang, M., & Stufken, J. (2019). Information-based optimal subdata selection for big data linear regression. *Journal of the American Statistical Association, 114*(525), 393–405.

White, L. V. (1973). An extension of the general equivalence theorem to nonlinear models. *Biometrika, 60*(2), 354–348.

Whittle, P. (1973). Some general points in the theory of optimal experimental design. *Journal of the Royal Statistical Society Series B, 35*, 123–130.

Wiens, D. P. (1991). Designs for approximately linear regression: Two optimality properties of uniform designs. *Statistics & Probability Letters, 12*, 217–221.

Wiens, D. P. (2019). Maximin power designs in testing lack of fit. *Journal of Statistical Planning and Inference, 119*, 311–317.

Wong, W. K., & Zhou, J. (2019). CVX-based algorithms for constructing various optimal regression designs. *Canadian Journal of Statistics-Revue Canadienne de Statistique, 47*(3), 374–391.

Wong, W. K., & Zhou, J. (2023). Using CVX to construct optimal designs for biomedical studies with multiple objectives. *Journal of Computational and Graphical Statistics, 32*(2), 744–753.

Wong, W. K. (1993). Minimal number of support-points for mini-max optimal designs. *Statistics & Probability Letters, 17*(5), 405–409.

Woods, D. C., Biedermann, S. & Tommasi, C. (Eds.). (2023). *mODa 13: Model-oriented data analysis and optimum design.* Stat Papers (in press).

Wu, Ch.-F., & Wynn, H. P. (1978). The convergence of general step-length algorithms for regular optimum design criteria. *The Annals of Statistics, 6*(6), 1273–1285.

Wynn, H. P. (1970). The sequential generation of D-Optimum experimental designs. *Annals of Mathematical Statistics, 41*(5), 1655–1664.

Yang, M., Biedermann, S., & Tang, E. (2013). On optimal designs for nonlinear models: A general and efficient algorithm. *Journal of the American Statistical Association, 108*(504), 1411–1420.

Ying, Z. (1993). Maximum likelihood estimation of parameters under a spatial sampling scheme. *The Annals of Statistics, 21*(3), 1567–1590.

Yu, W., Zhou, H., Choi, Y., Goldin, J. G., Teng, P., Wong, W. K., McNitt-Gray, M. F., Brown, M. S., & Kim, G. H. J. (2023). Multi-scale, domain knowledge-guided attention plus random forest: A two-stage deep learning-based multi-scale guided attention models to diagnose idiopathic pulmonary fibrosis from computed tomography images. *Medical Physics, 50*(2), 894–905.

Yu, Y. (2010). Monotonic convergence of a general algorithm for computing optimal designs. *Annals of Statistics, 38*(3), 1593–1606.

Zhu, Z., & Stein, M. L. (2005). Spatial sampling design for parameter estimation of the covariance function. *Journal of Statistical Planning and Inference, 134*, 583–603.

Zhu, Z., & Zhang, H. (2006). Spatial sampling design for parameter estimation of the covariance function. *Environmetrics, 17*, 323–337.

Index

J. López-Fidalgo, *Optimal Experimental Design*, Lecture Notes in Statistics 226,
https://doi.org/10.1007/978-3-031-35918-7

Printed in the United States
by Baker & Taylor Publisher Services